COUNSELLING IN MEDICAL SETTINGS

Patricia East

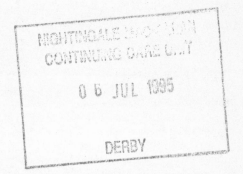

OPEN UNIVERSITY PRESS
Buckingham · Philadelphia

Open University Press
Celtic Court
22 Ballmoor
Buckingham
MK18 1XW

and
1900 Frost Road, Suite 101
Bristol, PA 19007, USA

First Published 1995

A catalogue record of this book is available from the British Library

ISBN 0 335 19241 6 (pb)

Library of Congress Cataloging-in-Publication Data
East, Patricia, 1944–
Counselling in medical settings / Patricia East.
p. cm. — (Counselling in context)
Includes bibliographical references and index.
ISBN 0–335–19241–6 (pbk.)
1. Mental health counseling. 2. Health counseling. 3. Primary
care (Medicine) 4. Mental health counseling—Great Britain.
5. Health counseling—Great Britain. 6. Primary care (Medicine)—
Great Britain. I. Title. II. Series.
[DNLM: 1. Counseling—methods. WM 55 E13c 1995]
RC466.E26 1995
362.1'04256—dc20
DNLM/DLC
for Library of Congress 94–40669
CIP

Typeset by Graphicraft Typesetters Ltd., Hong Kong
Printed in Great Britain by St Edmundsbury Press Ltd
Bury St Edmunds, Suffolk

COUNSELLING IN
MEDICAL SETTINGS

· COUNSELLING IN CONTEXT ·

Series editors
Moira Walker and Michael Jacobs
University of Leicester

Counselling takes place in many different contexts: in voluntary and statutory agencies; in individual private practice or in a consortium; at work, in medical settings, in churches and in different areas of education. While there may be much in common in basic counselling methods (despite theoretical differences), each setting gives rise to particular areas of concern, and often requires specialist knowledge, both of the problems likely to be brought, but also of the context in which the client is being seen. Even common counselling issues vary slightly from situation to situation in the way they are applied and understood.

This series examines eleven such areas, and applies a similar scheme to each, first looking at the history of the development of counselling in that particular context; then at the context itself, and how the counsellor fits into it. Central to each volume are chapters on common issues related to the specific setting and questions that may be peculiar to it but could be of interest and value to counsellors working elsewhere. Each book will provide useful information for anyone considering counselling, or the provision of counselling in a particular context. Relationships with others who work in the same setting whether as counsellors, managers or administrators are also examined; and each book concludes with the author's own critique of counselling as it is currently practised in that context.

Current and forthcoming titles

Elsa Bell: *Counselling in Further and Higher Education*
Judith Brearley: *Counselling and Social Work*
Dilys Davies: *Counselling in Psychological Services*
Patricia East: *Counselling in Medical Settings*
David Lyall: *Counselling in the Pastoral and Spiritual Context*
John Brazier: *Counselling at Work*
Janet Perry: *Counselling for Women*
Gabrielle Syme: *Counselling in Independent Practice*
Nicholas Tyndall: *Counselling in the Voluntary Sector*
Brian Williams: *Counselling in the Penal System*
Judith Mabey and Bernice Sorensen: *Counselling for Young People*

Contents

Series editors' preface

It is instructive to remind ourselves that Freud addressed his only writing on psychoanalytic technique to physicians. Counselling is not psychoanalysis, but its origins lie in that innovatory therapy, and indeed in medical circles. Freud himself, of course, did not wish to confine the practice of the talking therapy to doctors. He argued and wrote in defence of lay analysis. That example is one which in Britain especially we have much to be thankful for, because psychotherapy and counselling has not been reserved for the domain of either doctors or psychologists.

That there should now be counsellors in general practice might amaze those early pioneers, even those who laid aside their white coats and stethoscopes in favour of total engagement with the psychological. Doctors at their best, especially in general practice, have always known that the psyche is as important as the body, and that emotions and relationships are just as likely to be the trouble as anything physical. Whether it is another expression of the fashionable trends, or genuine conviction of the usefulness of talk and time; or whether it is a belief that it is cheaper than a mounting drugs bill, or the pressure that is coming from their patients, more and more practices are taking the opportunity to employ their own counsellors.

The editors and the author of this book, all have experience of working in the context of the National Health Service. Developments in primary care presently compensate somewhat for the cuts in services in many hospital departments. There is much to be welcomed, especially for those of us who were ourselves pioneers in the experiments that brought together medical staff and counsellors in common care of the same group of patients. There were problems then, often of understanding the pressures and expectations upon each profession, and there are bound to be problems now. Counsellors are no more a magical solution than any of the wonder drugs that pharmaceutical representatives peddle at the end of busy surgeries. Doctors may recommend counselling in desperation. Nurses may resent that much of their caring and conversational role has been encroached upon by practice counsellors. Each part of a general practice or a hospital department has its sacred territory. There is bound to be some envy of what the other professionals can offer – whether it be a prescription, an injection, or space to listen. Questions of confidentiality, of contracts and of confidence are perhaps even more pressing now, given both the demands of the work, but also the stronger position in which the counselling profession finds itself. It is no longer individual doctors, nurses and counsellors who pave the way. Counselling is now a major professional concern.

These and many other issues are raised in this book. The author applies her sharp and quizzical mind to counselling in medical settings as one who has been part of that scene, but who also stands outside it. This is a distinct advantage in writing about this setting, since the medical profession can sometimes take itself too seriously, conscious as it is of its importance to so many people. Not that Patricia East's treatment is less than serious itself, but it brings a freshness and an appropriate degree of questioning to the confluence of these two major professional activities. It is a book which merits being read by all who work in the National Health Service and in private medicine, both as a diagnostic tool and as a prophylactic measure wherever and whenever counsellors, para-medical and other staff and doctors share the same setting.

Moira Walker
Michael Jacobs

Preface and acknowledgements

These are important and challenging times for counsellors in medical settings. Questions about the incorporation of counselling as a distinct and separate healing process within this context inevitably highlight for the medical profession major issues of ethics, accountability, effectiveness, appropriateness and cost. Many counsellors in turn question how appropriately the counselling process fits within the medical model. Since there is no ideal state with which the outcome of counselling can be compared, counsellors use the notions of treatment and cure in a different way. Illnesses are part of peoples' life stories, part of their whole story not just the bit about their limbs or their organs but their whole beings in the context of their whole lives, even if during the course of an illness the person might feel isolated and alienated. This is the starting place for counselling in medical settings.

There is a good deal of discussion about counselling in medical settings and the way that it has developed in the following account, but this gives only a broad overview of this enormously complex and diverse provision. I have tried, as in the counselling process itself, to go beyond description and factual content and to get in touch with some of the feelings that are aroused in this particular context by including personal accounts from counsellors and their clients. I have been able to do this because I have been privileged in the writing of the book to have the support and encouragement of those who appear in it as representatives of the growing number of people involved in counselling in medical settings. I am grateful for their permission to re-tell their stories.

My thanks go to Dr Phil Hammond and Dr Tony Gardner, aka 'Struck Off and Die', for permission to use some of their material from 'Doctors with Attitudes'. Among the many counsellors and psychotherapists working in general practice who related their experiences to me, Annalee Curran and Marilyn Pietroni generously allowed me to quote them and then gave their time to review material and make useful suggestions. The late Viv Ball, as Vice-Chair of the Executive Committee of the Counselling in Medical Settings Division of the British Association for Counselling gave me a great deal of her time and support, contributing a valuable, personal insight into national developments in counselling in primary health care. Thanks are also due to Dr Glenys Parry, Senior Psychological Officer at the Mental Health, Elderly, Disability and Ethics Policy Branch at the Department of Health; Judith Baron and Robbi Campbell, who in addition to their respective roles as General Manager and Deputy Chair of BAC, are also counsellors in medical settings; Nancy Rowland from the Centre for Health Economics at the University of York; Professor David Wilkin at the Centre for Primary Care Research at the University of Manchester; Dr Tony Kendrick and Dr Andre Tylee from the Division of General Practice and Primary Care at St George's Hospital Medical School at the University of London; Dr Graham Curtis Jenkins, Director of the Counselling in Primary Care Trust; Patricia Fitzgerald, Counselling and Mental Health Advisor for Derbyshire FHSA; Jennifer Hunt, Counsellor at the Institute of Obstetrics and Gynaecology at Hammersmith Hospital; and Bill Barnes and Dr Michael Göpfert of the Liverpool Psychotherapy and Consultation Service.

I am grateful to all of the counsellors and clients who appear under their pseudonyms for their permission to use their stories. In particular, my thanks go to 'Verity', 'Su', 'Gilbert', 'Connor' and 'Darwin' for providing extensive and detailed examples of their counselling practice. Thanks also to the five medical students from the North-East and to the members of a Community Mental Health Team based in the East Midlands for their full and frank responses to my questionnaire survey about their experiences of counselling within their training and practice.

I am also grateful that I have been allowed to use material from other sources. All extracts have been reprinted with permission. The extract from *Out of the Doll's House* by Angela Holdsworth is reproduced with the permission of BBC Enterprises Ltd; the extracts from MIND's *Policy Pack* and Daphne Wood's *Wordswordswordswords, the Power of Words: Uses and Abuses of Talking Treatments* are reproduced with the permission of MIND Publications; and the extracts from the British Association for Counselling Publications with the permission of BAC. Please note that readers should check with the

BAC for any modifications to their codes, which may be made following the date of publication.

My final and special thanks go to Michael Jacobs and Moira Walker for believing that I had a book in me; to Moira for her patience and encouragement as editor during its preparation; to Sam Yates for preparing the manuscript with her usual style and efficiency; but most of all to my partner Roger Ellis who has sustained me throughout the whole experience.

· ONE ·

The development of counselling in medical settings

Advertisements for posts as counsellors in medical settings have begun to appear regularly in the national press and we are becoming accustomed to media reports of counselling being offered to people who have suffered trauma and loss. When it is woven seamlessly into the storyline of 'The Archers', the longest running radio serial, we realize the extent to which counselling is becoming integrated and accepted as part of everyday life. Since the inception of the Counselling in Medical Settings (CMS) Division of the British Association for Counselling (BAC) in 1977 there has been a growth (some would say an explosion) in the development of counselling in medical settings, although the provision nationally is patchy and varied. It is an appropriate time therefore to examine some of the basic issues that arise from this expansion and answer some questions about the counsellors and their clients, how they interface with other medical provision, what sort of problems they deal with and how effective they are. We will begin our examination in the most traditional and medically appropriate manner with a history of the subject, starting with a broad overview of how medicine itself has developed. Such an explanation is central to our understanding of the development of counselling within this context – a recent aspect of this history.

HISTORICAL OVERVIEW

Seale and Pattison (1994) offer an historical approach to medical knowledge which demonstrates that our views on medicine are inseparable from our culture and time. What we take for granted can be challenged when we visit another country or look back on what was done in the past in the name of medical treatments in our own country. Also, looking back to the past within our own culture explains how our present assumptions and practice developed and indicates a need to be more poised and sceptical about the validity of current treatments, some of which might well be viewed as strange, or even barbaric, in the future.

The development of ideas about how we respond to people who are ill or in need of medical attention is also a product of all aspects of our culture. Ethnic and cultural factors have been shown to influence people's responses to illness and their recognition of a need to consult a doctor (Corney and Jenkins 1993). It is not so many years ago that women in particular were too embarrassed to present their bodies for medical inspection; in some cultural groups this may still be the case. That most natural state of pregnancy was concealed by voluminous clothes until well into the middle of the twentieth century. Holdsworth (1988) relates the story of a woman who died at the age of 32 from septicaemia brought on by infected piles because she had been too shy to confide in a doctor.

Philosophical, religious, moral, intellectual, social, economic and political ideas have no inherent coherence or progression and many different and contradictory ideas can coexist at any one time. Even today, both lay people and competent medical practitioners draw on diverse and alternative views such as divine retribution and social deviance (in explanations for AIDS for example), possession by spirits, astrology or the weather (as in Seasonal Affective Disorder) to account for *dis-ease* in people. Another persistent view is that good health is linked to virtuous behaviour and ill health to general and deserved misfortune. There are clear links here with the stigmatizing effect of mental illness, hence the need for some people to explain *dis-ease* and mental pain as a physical illness which is somehow more acceptable. These various explanations have gripped the human imagination throughout history and persist in the face of, or possibly as more satisfying explanations than, modern medical knowledge.

The dominant paradigm in our present day culture, used to gain valid and reliable knowledge about medicine, is the scientific method which was originally applied to the investigation of the world of inanimate objects. A paradigm is an influential set of ideas, normally coherent and consistent, about the way the world or an aspect of the world operates. This world view, or frame of reference, tends to exclude or discredit alternative views, at least for a time (Kuhn 1962). In the context of this chapter it is relevant to ask how the dominance of the scientific research paradigm has come about and what alternative views have been and still tend to be excluded, discredited and devalued by those who are committed to the supremacy of this view of science. Seale and Pattison (1994) describe the development of this dominant paradigm alongside lay and traditional views of medicine.

LAY MEDICINE

Any understanding of the links between medicine and society and medicine and culture has to acknowledge the significance of lay care which is usually ministered by women to their families or by close relatives and friends. Until about the middle of the eighteenth century most diseases were treated by lay care in the home. Knowledge of medical treatments was much more widely owned. There was a consensus that the whole person, physically, emotionally and spiritually, was involved in his or her own disease, illness and health. Before the advent of free health care this was all that many could afford and it was culturally acceptable as part of women's role that they delivered babies, cared for the sick and laid out the dead. My own Aunty Annie was often fetched out to help someone in our street. Annie had trained as a nurse and had served in France in World War I. She appeared to spend her entire life in a cotton wraparound pinny with a bottle of sal volatile tucked in the pocket. Aunty Annie was always available to deliver a baby, lay out a body and generally dispense a good deal of common sense and reassurance by her mere presence. With the advent of the free National Health Service (NHS) such care became increasingly medicalized as many people, especially women, visited their local doctor for the first time. However, only a small percentage of minor illnesses are treated by doctors. Local pharmacies supply an enormous number of preparations over their counters to treat everything from headaches to athlete's foot. It is likely that a good deal of support is also offered, largely unrecognized, in response to emotional distress and pain.

Historically, the lay treatment of people with mental abnormalities has been dealt with in a variety of non-medical ways. If they hurt or frightened other people they might be burned or stoned, imprisoned, exploited and degraded. If they mystified and amused they might be held in awe, honoured, and respected. And if they were taken seriously then they might have received, or suffered, a variety of treatments, often based on religious, superstitious or magical beliefs. As knowledge and understanding grew, the gap widened between medical practice and religion and superstition. Witchcraft, sorcery and possession by devils were once used to explain misfortune and illness. Germs, bacteria, pollution, radiation and the stress of modern society are often used as the contemporary equivalents of these evil spirits. Social factors such as poor housing, unemployment and the breakdown of families are also used to explain illnesses, though personal thoughts, fears and fantasies might still draw on different and more primitive explanations. Authors such as Susan Sontag (1978; 1991) and, more recently, Michael Ignatieff (1994) have both written expressively about the ways that diseases such as AIDS, cancer and Alzheimer's disease are first identified with and then become metaphors for the dark and fearful side of human experience.

We have a need to explain pain, to make sense of the experience, to account for the meaning of illness. A diagnosis of a disease by a doctor might contrast with the lay person's view of having an illness. Illnesses are experiences with personal meaning, diseases are abnormalities which have recognized structures and development. It is possible to have a disease without feeling ill and to feel ill without having a disease, (which does not mean the same thing as 'there's nothing wrong with you'). Doctors and nurses may recognize the factors which contribute to distress and pain from their professional viewpoint and prescribe and deliver sensitive and appropriate care. At the same time, their lay beliefs may offer them more personal, non-professional interpretations which might affect their behaviour towards people in their care. There is, for example, sometimes an ambivalence in the treatment and care of people who have self-harmed if they are viewed as wasting time and resources that could, in the carer's opinion, be better spent on others more deserving. It also happens that when staff are dealing with their own distress they sometimes fall back on self-blame and private moralities which are more firmly rooted in their lay beliefs than in a rational understanding of medicine. The work of counsellors in medical settings, in addition to dealing with clients' needs to make sense, or come to terms with the personal experience of illness, can also involve helping staff to handle ambivalence and the tension and conflict it arouses.

TRADITIONAL MEDICINE

Historically, this holistic view took account of the way that an individual's constitution and personal habits interacted with cosmic influences and the local environment. The humoral theory of the Greeks was a totally interactive explanation of disease which was seen as the result of disharmony between nature and supernature. The idealized Greek physician, Hippocrates (c. 460–357 BC), known as the father of medicine, followed the dominant paradigm of his time, the doctrine of the four bodily humours, which guided medical thinking for many centuries. The body was viewed as a microcosm of the universe, composed of the four elements of nature: fire, air, earth and water. An individual's constitution was reckoned to be determined by the relative proportions of the four chief bodily fluids, or cardinal humours: blood (sanguine); phlegm (phlegmatic); yellow bile (choleric); and black bile (melancholic), and the way that these interacted with the physical conditions of hot/cold and dry/wet. Therapeutic treatments were aimed at correcting any perceived imbalance. Hippocrates believed that our natures are the physicians of our diseases and refuted the idea that disease was a punishment from the gods, noting instead the effects of diet, occupation and climate.

Traditional treatments such as 'washouts', which are still popular with some ethnic groups as a total body-cleansing process, and the belief that hot drinks cure colds are examples of present day applications of these ideas. There are still vestiges of this way of thinking in our everyday language and descriptions of people's feelings about their health and well-being. Blood, bile, and phlegm are used in evocative ways, especially when linked with their traditional elemental and physical counterparts, to describe feelings and temperaments. George Eliot (1871) in her novel *Middlemarch* portrays the epitome of a dry character in Edward Casaubon.

Traditional treatments are offered by specialist healers such as acupuncturists, herbalists and masseurs. Both the longevity and current growth in popularity and demand for these treatments are a testament to their place in the range of provision. They are viewed as non-orthodox by our scientific, bio-medical standards but as orthodox and mainstream in other cultures. The growing recognition of such traditional methods gained government support in the House of Commons when, in February 1994, an unopposed second reading of a Bill to enforce the registration of chiropractors led to a widening of the issue to include support for all complementary practices.

THE SCIENTIFIC MEDICAL MODEL

The Doctors' Registration Act of 1858 had many consequences. Research began to expand, using the bodies of the poor; an accepted programme of training and education started to become established, and the consequent power and prestige of doctors eventually became encoded in new textbooks. The scientific method became the dominant paradigm with emphasis on analysis and on the new tools of identification and classification and the assumption of cause and effect in detecting underlying pathology. Medical specialization inevitably began, particularly with regard to training and treatments. The patient began to be seen as a carrier of a disease in contrast to both lay and traditional medicine in which the whole person was considered as an expression of the disease. An inevitable consequence of the application of the scientific method, with its fundamental value of reductionism, was that the body was viewed as a machine and clinical medicine became mechanistic.

No one today can know all there is to know about medicine. Just as science itself developed from the root layering of philosophy to produce vigorous new independent offshoots, so medical knowledge has branched out into its own specialist areas. Philosophy and medicine both began with a holistic perception of the person. Both found their way to compartmentalization, minds separated off from bodies. When Freud discovered the unconscious he was still a biologist, a biologist of the mind. His earliest ideas fitted the dominant mechanistic, scientific theories of the time. Freud's ambition was to claim a scientific pedigree for psychoanalysis. The social sciences also adopted the rules of the physical sciences in order to be accepted as intellectually rigorous and respectable. To a large extent they are still governed by them, while inexorably science itself has moved forward. Radical ideas from physics this century have fundamentally challenged the historical split of mind and body by questioning the basic distinction of observer and observed, resulting in a shift in the philosophical basis of science itself. It is now much more respectable to hold an interactionist view of mind and body. With that, the holistic view of the person becomes central once again. Of course, many non-scientists have never had a problem with these ideas, and developments in traditional and lay medicine have always taken just such a holistic, interactionist view. The current debate about the necessity and effectiveness of the talking treatments, compared with scientific medical treatments, tends to create rivalrous opposition between the two views. This opposition may inhibit investigations into their complementary nature and promote an avoidance of the potentially creative aspects of uncertainty. Paradoxically, three central ideas of twentieth-century physics – complementarity, relativity and uncertainty – are also central to counselling and psychotherapy.

The strength of the scientific medical model is attributable to empiricism which demands actual investigation to identify and consequently explain phenomena. From the sixteenth century it became increasingly possible to investigate anatomy through dissection rather than speculation. Psychological investigations are obviously not accessible to this type of exploration and understanding and if this is seen as the only valid method, approaches that cannot be 'proved' in this way will inevitably appear questionable. This does not make them invalid but it does mean that alternative methods of investigation will be challenged and need to be expanded and developed. The debate about the body–mind distinction is still very much alive and is central to the drugs versus counselling issues because it centres on what counts as valid proof of effectiveness in medicine. The massive development of laboratory medicine to support clinical work has strengthened the scientific paradigm as the norm against which other methods are compared. Research into the effectiveness of counselling in medical settings has to meet demands for scientific rigour (King 1994; King *et al.* 1994). There are also vested interests. Not only is there a struggle between intellectual paradigms, but considerable commercial interest exists. For example, drug companies employ a huge number of staff in their own and allied medical research and can build the cost of this into the price of their products. Research into the effectiveness of counselling and psychotherapy has never had comparable funding and personnel even though there are persistent demands for such research.

HEALING THE PSYCHE: A BRIEF HISTORY

There are huge gaps in our knowledge about how people were dealt with in medical settings up until about 200 years ago. Psychiatry and psychotherapy and the talking treatments are relatively young branches of medicine, though the problems and issues they address are as old as the human race itself. Mental pathology, symptoms and behaviour, have always been recognized and described in literature if not in medical tracts.

'In sooth, I know not why I am so sad', says Antonio at the beginning of the *Merchant of Venice*, appealing to his friends in his need to find solace for his feelings. If he presented his feelings to a GP today he might, depending on the orientation and resources available to the doctor, be prescribed an anti-depressant drug or be referred to a practice counsellor. The GP would know, if at all interested in statistics, and certainly from experience, that his unhappy

patient was one of many thousands of people who present annually
to their doctors with feelings of depression and anxiety.

For as long as people have had feelings they have had sad, bad
and mad feelings alongside their happier states of mind. The oldest
known written record is probably the *Dialogue of a Life Weary Man
with his Soul*, an Egyptian account of the psychology of suicide from
about 2000 BC. The healers of ancient civilizations, the medicine
men and women, or shamans, used their own charismatic personalities developed over a lengthy and arduous training and initiation
period during their treatments. Their powers, though often claimed
as magical, were essentially psychological.

From prehistory to the middle ages, when a person was understood to be possessed by evil spirits, primitive cures ranged from
stoning to exorcism and trepanning, whereby a hole was drilled
into the skull in order to release the spirits. Less drastic measures
included the use of herbs and plants; rauwolfia, for example, has
been used as a tranquillizer for a thousand years. Critics of modern
mental health treatments could claim that we have not progressed
very far, citing the continued use of electroconvulsive therapy (ECT)
and psychotropic drugs, with their unpleasant and debilitating side
effects (Breggin 1993).

A more positive example of practice in psychological healing is
that of Asclepius, the mythical Greek god of medicine, in whose
honour hundreds of shrines and temples were built, the remains of
which can still be seen in Athens and Cos. These shrines, called
Asclepeia, attracted many pilgrims seeking cures. They were built in
beautiful, prestigious places where people could undertake purifica-
tion rites. One of these rites was the incubation, a night's sleep in
the temple dormitory on a couch or on the ground. This was undertaken in the hope that the person might experience *epiphamia*, a
healing process including a therapeutic dream, in which Asclepius,
or one of his priests would appear to deliver a message or advice,
thus revealing the solution to personal problems.

Throughout history there is evidence that 'talking treatments'
have been used to relieve psychic pain and suffering, even if the
dominant ethos was on self-control rather than on insight or expression of feelings. The Stoics, a school of Greek philosophers
founded in about 300 BC, believed in control of the emotions, and
promoted an austere indifference to pleasure and pain and a patient
endurance of suffering. Another founding father of medicine,
Claudius Galen (*c.* AD 130–200), writing 'On the Passions of the
Soul', described how, with the help of a wise mentor to point out
faults and give sound advice, patients attained serenity and freedom

from emotional responses until eventually they were able to help others in the same way. Therapy *by the word* was an aspect of the Cathartic, Dialectic and Rhetorical dialogues of the Greeks and their patients. The *consolation*, a therapeutic dialogue which could be written or spoken, was encouraged and frequently used. This could be a letter, sometimes a poem, written to help a patient recover a peaceful state of mind, for example, following a bereavement. An example of this is the consolation letter that Plutarch wrote to his wife following the death of their child. Perhaps letters have always been used by friends and relatives to offer consolation and support. A more formal use of the letter as a therapeutic intervention can be recognized today in Cognitive Analytic Therapy (CAT) (see p. 44). There are also similarities between another ancient idea and some modern cognitive and behavioural therapies used to treat people who have problems with alcohol abuse. In the Middle Ages, Rhazes, a Persian doctor dealing with drunkenness and its causes in his book, *The Spiritual Physik of Rhazes*, recommended a talking treatment to dispel anxiety and replace it with courage and cheerfulness.

Some mental hospitals built in the thirteenth century were luxurious. The hospital in Cairo contained fountains, summer and winter rooms, was furnished with fine silk cushions, and offered treatments combining drug, music and perfume therapies. Much more common are descriptions of hospitals with harsh conditions and treatments. The growth of Christianity promoted the role of caring for the sick, and infirmaries were opened in large monasteries. Confession and absolving of sins often involved excessive penitential behaviours. However, alongside punitive and superstitious exorcisms and suggestive healing, an enlightened form of care in the community for the mentally ill was established at Gheel in Belgium in the thirteenth century. This is still in existence today, with people who are mentally ill fully integrated into the everyday life of the town.

With the development of the printing press in the fifteenth century more detailed medical information became available. The study of melancholia was of particular interest throughout Europe. Robert Burton's *The Anatomy of Melancholy*, published in 1621, described the various aspects of melancholia as a 'labyrinth of doubts and errors'. Melancholia became a fashionable condition in England and its characteristic states of moodiness, bitter irony, eccentricity, misanthropy, a general disgust with life and predisposition to suicide, were described as being typically English!

When Freud (1856–1939) introduced the world to psychoanalysis over a hundred years ago, he revolutionized its understanding of the unconscious, using rational thought to explain the irrational. However, there were many observations of unconscious activities before Freud. Descartes' story of falling in love with a cock-eyed woman, whom he subsequently connected with a similar love from his childhood, reinforced his view that unexplained feelings and aversions could be traced back to the forgotten events of childhood, which, if remembered, would stop the pain in the present. But there was no extrapolation from this by Descartes, or any of his contemporaries, into the field of human healing. Priest and ministers still offered comfort by relieving people of the burden of their guilty secrets. John Wesley (1703–91) the English preacher and founder of Methodism is reputed to have had a profound understanding of emotional problems, while the Quakers, members of a religious society founded by George Fox in 1648–50, applied their peaceful principles to work with the insane and mentally ill well before such a humane response was commonly accepted. Imprisonment, whether in a monastery or a prison, became the widely used response to fools who were chained up alongside criminals and beggars.

Depression has traditionally been linked with sin, and healing linked with confession, atonement and reconciliation with the gods. The Psalms of David, which are central to the Judaic–Christian tradition, provide us with many examples of this. Today, when we say, 'I feel bad' when feeling ill, the dual meaning of illness and badness may be conveyed. Our ideas about illness, our moral codes, beliefs and values affect our ability to seek help. If depression is linked with badness it leads to shame and guilt, the stigma being made worse by the underlying feeling that somehow the person is responsible. This might express itself in self-harm or be disguised as a more acceptable physical symptom. Psychosomatic presentations are discussed in more detail in Chapter 4.

People who had problems that were not straightforward and easily understood, especially if they frightened others or contravened existing social norms, were shut away for long periods, sometimes for their whole lives. Deviance from what was considered normal included pregnancy outside marriage (interpreted as a symptom of promiscuity and wayward behaviour) and post-natal depression. This happened in the case of one young woman, Rose, who was admitted to a psychiatric hospital in 1960 suffering from post-natal depression following the birth of her third child and who became separated and isolated as she lost contact with her family. Rose remained in hospital for the next 30 years. More recently, changes in attitudes and policies have led to the closure of large mental hospitals and many people like Rose have started to rebuild their lives in the community, but for many years the solution – to allay individual fears and incorporate widespread denial and repression – was to remove the person of from the eyes of the wider society and thus from its conscious awareness. This splitting off and consequent hiding away of frightening aspects of humanity resonated with the dominant dualistic thinking that was the basis of scientific medical thinking, leading to a simplistic and unsophisticated dichotomy of

body	_____	mind
ill	_____	well
unhealthy	_____	healthy
patients	_____	medical staff

rather than an understanding and appreciation of health as a complex and dynamic equilibrium. To counteract such splitting it is necessary that the patient be taken seriously as a whole person which, in turn, requires that she or he be listened to with care and commitment. The ability to listen to patients and accurately diagnose underlying conditions will be a theme throughout the following chapters. In the 1950s this became the focus of Michael Balint's work with general practitioners.

MICHAEL BALINT: THE DOCTOR–PATIENT RELATIONSHIP

It was the need to integrate a comprehensive understanding of the patient's presenting problem that led Michael Balint, whose father had been a general practitioner, to begin his work with GPs. Balint was an analyst and disciple of the Hungarian psychoanalyst Sandor Ferenczi. A contemporary of Freud, Ferenczi was influential in the development of psychoanalytical thinking which emphasized the importance of interpersonal relationships. Balint's use of selected analytic concepts with GPs was an extension of his psychoanalytic work and an example of his fertile and creative application of these ideas into allied areas. Collaboration with his first wife, Alice, whose interest in comparative pedagogics during the 1930s had led to her seminal work on the mother–infant relationship, contributed towards Balint's later theories about the ways that people relate to themselves, to others and to their environment. This early work also led to an increased awareness and understanding of the importance of the therapist's own emotional responsiveness to a person as an essential component of the therapeutic process. This in turn

contributed to a growing understanding and awareness of the significance of the therapist's affective response, what in psychodynamic
therapy and counselling has come to be valued as that part of the
therapeutic exchange known as the therapist's counter transference.

Balint used his psychoanalytic training and understanding to help
GPs better understand their patients' needs. With his second wife
Enid, he organized seminars for GPs to study their work with patients. The Balints' emphasis was to focus attention on the doctor's
relationship with the patient. In *The Doctor, His Patient and the Illness*
(Balint, M. 1957) and in *Six Minutes for the Patient* (Balint and Norell
1973) they describe how GPs can become participant observers of
their own practice in order to make more insightful responses to
their patients' presenting problems. Guided initially by Balint and
then by other seminar leaders who were usually psychoanalysts,
groups of practising doctors were encouraged to explore new methods and techniques of working with their patients. These were not
therapy groups. The focus remained firmly on the doctor–patient
relationship, the objective being to enable GPs to clarify their observations and to engage with their patients at a meaningful emotional
level within a few minutes of consultation. As 'sovereign masters of
their own surgeries' Balint believed that GPs were ideally placed to
deal with patients' emotional responses to their diseases, being able
to draw upon a wealth of background knowledge and information
with which to complement their medical understanding. A recent
re-evaluation of Balint's work points out the disadvantages of working as a counsellor without this rich background. (Balint, E. *et al.*
1993). Although the number of Balint groups has declined since the
1970s, his work in developing what he called research-training
seminars with small groups of doctors has been adapted and continued by other group facilitators in this country, Germany and the
USA.

A NATIONAL HEALTH SERVICE

The physicist Richard Feynman (1918–88) said that Nature uses the
longest threads to weave her patterns and, even from this brief
introduction, the reader will see that throughout the history of
medicine the connection between body and mind has been a long
and interweaving thread which has been variously understood and
variously treated. The question now arises of how this history relates to modern times and modern thinking and its particular relevance for the development of counselling in medical settings.

With the introduction of the National Health Service (1948) general practitioners became independent contractors within the new Service, 80 per cent of them working single-handed, their contracts administered by executive councils. At the same time the development of institutional medicine, including the major teaching hospitals, added to the hope for medicine that was linked to the ideals of socialism and the welfare state – free medicine and treatment for everyone. The numbers of women consulting a doctor increased dramatically and, as Dr John Fry noted from records maintained over 40 years in order to examine the medical profile of women, 'as physical ailments lessened, psychological ones became more apparent' (Holdsworth 1988:105). Evidence such as this highlights the contextual importance of psychological problems. One result was an alarming rise in the numbers and amount of drugs prescribed to deal with what was often a complex social, emotional and physical problem.

The 1950s was a difficult decade for family doctors. They became detached from hospital services and, since any money spent on their practices had to come from their own income, little was invested in practices. General Practice probably felt like Cinderella without a fairy godmother. District nurses and health visitors were frequently separated from GPs; there was little direct communication or coherent care, and many doctors resisted nurses being attached to their practices, being unclear about their roles and qualifications and defensive about their own territory and ownership of patients. This is reflected in the findings of a Royal College of General Practitioners Survey in 1964 which found little interest in preventative care (Hasler 1993). Many doctors had little knowledge or understanding of health visitors' qualifications and skills and, communications with nursing staff were often poor. This picture of initial ambivalence towards nurses and health visitors and resistance to their incorporation into general practice can be compared with the more recent introduction of counsellors into this setting.

THE EMERGENCE OF THE PRIMARY HEALTH CARE TEAM

The formation of the Royal College of Practitioners in 1952 brought together the influence of powerful minds and spirits to work towards increasing the professional status of the GP and to encourage a team approach to primary health care. Primary care is about the initial contact between GPs and their patients, the co-ordination of that contact when referrals are made to other members of the health care team and to consultants or specialists, and continued contact with patients and their families, often in a supportive and advisory role in addition to medical treatment. At first GPs were not enthusiastic about the College's recommendations. There was a conservative reaction as the doctors feared loss of power, authority and control. Less than half wanted health visitors attached to their practices.

Nursing in the United Kingdom in the 1950s was increasingly influenced by developments in the profession in the USA, which had shifted adherence from a medical model to an interpersonal relationship model, a movement which is still in progress. This meant that people's needs were increasingly being recognized as holistic rather than being reduced to a set of symptoms which could be diagnosed and treated. At much the same time that Balint was advocating the central role of the relationship between doctor and patient in general practice, an interpersonal model of nursing with contractual agreement between nurse and patient was being developed. This model enabled many nurses to develop and integrate their skills of listening and responding to patients' needs into their more traditional role, skills which would become increasingly identified as counselling skills.

The Family Doctors' Charter in 1966 stimulated the development of teamwork and encouraged the formation of group practices. Ancillary staff could now be employed with 70 per cent of their costs reimbursed by the local Health Authorities. The numbers of medical secretaries, receptionists and nurses employed by family doctors began to increase. The 70 per cent ancillary budget allowed for the first counsellors to be employed as part of primary health care (PHC) teams during this period. Doctors began to delegate tasks to the practice nurses, especially after the Health Service and Public Health Act allowed district nurses to treat patients in practice premises as well as in the patients' homes. Although the take-up of attached nurses had started slowly, their value was ultimately demonstrated by their work with patients. Nursing staff showed themselves particularly valuable in work that involved communication with patients, for example, in educating and in checking their understanding of care routines. In their work with chronically ill patients, nurses could offer appropriate follow-up and monitoring of chronic diseases such as asthma, diabetes and hypertension (Hasler 1993). Preventative work and health promotion also fell into their remit. This was not just a case of saving time but of making better use of the time of appropriate staff.

This was also a period when the different professional groups (the health visitors, district nurses, midwives and social workers) began to express their individual contributions and place within the PHC team. While, on the one hand, these groups valued their roles in the team and the improvement in communications between the different professional groups, on·the other they were concerned about losing their professional autonomy. Characteristic areas of their work, including counselling, might be submerged into medical treatment (Martin 1993). However, counselling as an integral part of PHC slowly became more established during the 1970s, both within the roles of existing staff and as an independent aspect of the team's range of provision.

By 1970, 75 per cent of health visitors and 68 per cent of district nurses were attached to general practices. General practitioners' contracts at this time were administered by Family Practitioner Committees (FPCs) This did not entirely solve issues of poor communication between doctors and other health care providers, nor did it resolve the variations and weaknesses in standards in primary care. Neglect of health promotion continued, as did lack of monitoring and control with little or no consumer involvement. Inner city areas and minority groups were disadvantaged, a situation that is still a cause for concern. The reorganization of the NHS in 1974 placed an increased emphasis on an integrated approach.

The first comprehensive review of Primary Health Care Services was undertaken a decade later, resulting in the publication of two reports in 1986, *Primary Health Care: An Agenda for Discussion* (DHSS 1986) and *Neighbourhood Nursing: A Focus for Care* (The Cumberlege Report) (DHSS 1986). The Cumberlege Report was commissioned to report on nursing services provided outside hospital in order to deploy resources more effectively to improve these services. When the views of nurses employed by GPs were explored they revealed feelings of isolation and being trapped by tradition. The review's findings were challenging for general practitioners, suggesting that nurses be recognized as professional equals and given shared responsibility. In spite of a negative response from general practitioners, who were particularly concerned about the employment status of practice nurses, the review initiated progress towards shifting community nursing services into general practice. Martin (1993) shows that although over 90 per cent of contact with patients took place in the community via primary care, this was 'processional' rather than integrated, with little evidence of quality teamwork, as people saw one professional after another. Martin's picture of a wheel of misfortune, with the patient as 'recipient of' rather than 'partner in' care does not include a specific reference to counsellors, assuming the counselling role to be part of other professional groups' activities rather than a distinct occupational area in its own right.

The increasing pressure to create a service responsive to the health care needs of the majority of the population is demonstrated in the central concerns of three government white papers published in the late 1980s. These were: *Promoting Better Health* (SSSS 1987); *Working for Patients* (SSSS 1989); and *Nursing in the Community* (NHS Management Executive 1990). The major thrust of *Promoting Better Health* was the promotion of good health and the implementation of a complete family health service rather than one which emphasized the treatment of disease. This was significant for the development of counselling in primary care because there was a specific recommendation to include counselling into an increased range of surgery services. The funding made available for increased and additional services facilitated the employment of counsellors.

Other recommendations included growth in preventative measures such as screening in pregnancy and for cervical cancer and new targets were set for vaccination and immunization. Well Woman and Well Man clinics were offered, along with other provision designed to raise awareness of the effects of diet and lifestyle on health. Clinics and support groups were started on How to prevent heart disease; Give-up smoking; and Manage stress to name but a few. Such health management clinics were able to generate income to support the employment of counsellors within general practices.

General practice acts as a gateway to hospitals or other specialist provision, often referred to as secondary health care. Except in the case of an accident or emergency and some specialist clinics, the family doctor is the patients' referral point. *Working for Patients* (SSSS 1989) recommended changes in the provision of secondary health care linked to separating the funding of health care from its provision. The budgets to purchase health care on behalf of NHS patients, or consumers would no longer be allocated to hospitals but to GPs or the District Health Authority. Treatment could be purchased from *any* provider. The intention of these reforms was to offer consumers more say in the range of services, a wider choice and more influence on how services would be provided.

By 1989, 80 per cent of family doctors were working in group practices with the trend towards bigger teams providing a variety of health care. As a result of these reforms many larger practices have become fund-holders. In addition to purchasing secondary health care, fund-holding practices have increased flexibility to purchase complementary treatments such as chiropody, physiotherapy, acupuncture and counselling or to employ staff to provide these services.

New contracts for GPs in 1990 further encouraged them to increase the amount and variety of their work. The FPCs became Family Health Service Authorities (FHSAs) offering financial incentives to support the government's increased emphasis on preventive and professional aspects of health care. The demands of setting budgets, the responsibility for auditing information with a growing reliance on information technology, and new contracting arrangements have all added to the management role of the family practitioner. For some this has been an opportunity to express entrepreneurial flair and has provided a new found freedom to deliver flexible and responsive medical care. For others it has been an enormous strain in terms of time, attention and personal values and preferred working focus, and an unwelcome distraction from an already fully-committed working life. Having the resources to employ additional staff has meant that some aspects of care and its management can be delegated. Opportunities for employing counsellors have been enhanced, if not yet embedded, into financial structures.

Nursing in the Community (NHS Management Executive 1990) urged the need for a collaborative approach between District Health Authorities (DHAs), FHSAs and local Social Services as purchasers and providers, with the emphasis on putting patients first. The success of such a joint venture will depend, according to the report, on a shared vision of care, joint assessments, and working together in a joint strategy with effective communications and commitment to quality. These themes will be further taken up in Chapter 5, but are emphasized by Sheppard:

> If general practitioners are to delegate specific tasks to other members of the team they must do so with a clear knowledge of their fellow professional's capabilities, a knowledge which includes awareness of the content of the training they have undertaken, so that there is no ambiguity about the limitations as well as the extent to which their role can reasonably be extended.
>
> (Sheppard 1993:68)

There are significant implications here for GPs considering employing practice counsellors and for the counsellor's role. As part of the Government's Citizens' Charter initiative, *The Patients' Charter* (detailing seven legal rights) was issued by the Department of Health in 1991. The Charter sets out the rights to care in the NHS, including the right of every citizen to receive health care based on clinical need regardless of ability to pay; to be registered with a GP; to receive emergency care; to be referred to a consultant; to be given a clear explanation of any proposed treatment; to have access to records; and to choose whether or not to take part in research or medical student training. The Charter also includes standards of service which are not legally binding. In 1992 an additional three legal patients' rights covering information on local health services, guaranteed admission dates and complaints procedures were added. Each DHA has followed up the national charter with its own interpretation and statement of local services to meet the required standards. The DHAs now have a duty to evaluate their services in terms of value for money, completion of contracts and maintenance/improvement of standards. The implications for accountability include, at least in theory, that the consumers views are considered. As a consequence there is an intention to progress towards the acceptance that doctors and patients are in partnership. As with the time lag between new medical discoveries and their wider application and acceptance, there may well be a gap between political rhetoric and actual change in attitudes and practice. A further analysis of this situation is made in Chapter 6.

THE INTRODUCTION OF COUNSELLING IN MEDICAL SETTINGS

Good quality health care is currently judged by a variety of outcome measures, some of which are more difficult to evaluate, especially as patients tend to be supportive of their carers even when they are not happy about the care they have received. The current scene is dominated by change. It is well recognized that the most powerfully conducive way to increase stress is to orchestrate as many changes as possible at the same time. Within a few years major structural changes in the NHS have resulted in the introduction of new contracts for GPs, radical changes in nurse education and training, Trust status for hospitals, fund-holding in general practice, a new policy on care in the community, and patients' charters and quality mechanisms. When organizations and structure are changed so rapidly and extensively it is not surprising that there are gaps and breakdowns in communication. For a profession that deals with mental and physical stress and consequent breakdown of human bodies there is sometimes an omnipotent denial of the stresses and trauma within its own organizational and institutional bodies which act to contain and define its work. This may

account for some of the resistances and difficulties that have confronted the development of counselling in medical settings.

To understand the current position of counselling in medical
settings it is necessary to understand something of the way that the
medical profession itself has evolved. One of the current and ongoing themes regarding counselling in medical settings is that doctors
do not understand what it is. In one sense history is repeating itself
since for many centuries there were no standardized job descriptions for doctors and nurses. Until the Medical Act of 1858 there
was no common medical register. As a result of the Act apothecar-
ies, physicians and surgeons merged to form a hospital-based service with a consequent agreement that physicians and surgeons would
treat patients referred from general practice. Primary care became
broadly-based and hospital care became increasingly specialized and
technical. Job descriptions for doctors were not produced until the
1960s and no standards were defined until the 1980s. Not until
1860, when the National School of Nurses opened at St Thomas'
Hospital, was the role of nurse defined. The 1948 statutory requirement for health visiting in the NHS specified that this be provided
by 'qualified women', leaving scope for wide-ranging interpretations.
The Council for the Training of Health Visitors was set up in 1902,
and a later development incorporated 'Education' into its title. There
was no mandatory requirement for education for district nurses
until 1981. The Nurses, Midwives and Health Visitors Act of 1979
established the United Kingdom Central Council for Nursing, Midwifery and Health Visiting (UKCC) which defines standards of training and professional conduct. *Project 2000: A New Preparation for Practice*
(UKCC 1986) introduced a new preparatory course for all nursing
students in which the nursing role is directed towards promoting
knowledgeable, reflective practitioners as nurses strive for professional status. The aim was to reform and modernize nurse education
and training making it more responsive to changing patterns of health
care at a time when demographic influences were indicating potential recruitment problems. Unless they had taken a personal initiative to become trained in counselling or counselling skills, nursing
staff who qualified before these reforms may have had no specific
training in this area. Project 2000 includes a module on counselling
skills within the course curriculum and opportunities for further
counselling training within the specialized vocational areas.

Project 2000 made a significant change in attitude and approach.
Prior to this nursing staff might have displayed varying degrees of
sensitivity and insight into their patients' feelings but *counselling* was
not a word commonly used in this country, particularly in the

medical profession, until relatively recently. From the 1960s counselling as a distinct process began to be increasingly recognized,
particularly through the work of client centred therapists, notably
Carl Rogers, in the United States. The Standing Conference for the
Advancement of Counselling (SCAC) was inaugurated in 1970 and
the British Association for Counselling (BAC) was founded from this
in 1977. However, as we shall see below, this was only the beginning
of what has come to be a major activity, in time filtering through
to long-standing professions such as medicine. There was already
enough interest and involvement in counselling in medical settings
by the 1970s for a separate Division within the newly formed BAC.

COUNSELLING IN MEDICAL SETTINGS
DIVISION OF BAC

The growth in membership of the Counselling in Medical Settings
(CMS) Division within the BAC since its inception in October 1977
signals a gradually increasing awareness and provision rather than
a sudden or recent development in this area. The history of the
CMS Division is characterized by a struggle to promote, develop and
maintain itself, which possibly reflects the struggle of the fledgling
counselling services which it seeks to support. The Executive members have always had a dual role as both architects and builders of
policies and guidelines. The Division counts as its two major achievements the establishment and maintenance of its newsletter and its
work on counselling in general practice. The CMS newsletter began
as a photocopied handout in 1984 and developed into a quarterly
journal. This is the Division's major networking instrument, a cohesive influence representing a membership which is geographically widespread and disparate in terms of occupational contexts,
roles and philosophies.

An apparent increase in counselling in general practice in the
early 1980s was noted by the CMS Division even though there was
a lack of evidence to substantiate it (Abel-Smith *et al.* 1989) and
little to guide employers and counsellors. As a result BAC established
a working party which met regularly between 1982–84 and led to
the publication of two guides. In 1985 *Counselling in General Practice:
A Guide for Counsellors* was first issued and in the same year '*Counselling in General Practice: A Guide For General Practitioners* was produced. Both guides have since been revised and reissued (Hurd and
Rowland 1991 revised edn, Irving and Heath 1989 revised edn).

In an effort to promote contact with its members after the lack of grass roots support made it impossible to hold the annual general meeting in 1985, the Division conducted a national survey of its members to find out more information about their wants, needs and interests, so that it could be more responsive and relevant. The survey revealed a strong sense of isolation amongst the membership of CMS. There were attempts to 'establish regional support groups as a consequence of these findings but on the whole these efforts were unsuccessful. The Executive settled for publication of a list of BAC branches in the CMS newsletter and the maintenance of a database of members. Similar results followed a second question- naire in 1990.

As its contribution to a Department of Health and Social Security review in 1986, CMS organized a survey on counselling in general practice through the FPCs (which later became FHSAs). This found that 28 FPCs had been contacted by doctors who were investigating possible routes for employing counsellors in their practices. Since there was no nationally agreed coherent system for appointing and paying counsellors then (or now) the survey is likely to have re- vealed only the tip of the iceberg.

BAC also sponsored a survey conducted by Glenys Breakwell in 1987 to map counselling provision in the NHS outside primary care. The survey was based on a national postal questionnaire survey of DHAs, professional associations and training bodies and an in-depth interview survey of a cross-section of staff. Breakwell aimed to discover where counsellors worked in the NHS outside the primary care sector. She looked at what was meant by counselling; when it was used; and how it was perceived as part of the work of those who were not primarily counsellors. This included a description of how counsellors were recruited, selected, inducted, trained and super- vised and/or supported. The object was to establish whether their job descriptions explicitly included their counselling activities; what position they occupied and their conditions of service. Breakwell also investigated what kinds of staff were regarded as having a counsel- ling element in their work: by themselves; by their colleagues or managers; and by their professional bodies or organizations.

Of the 200 questionnaires sent by Breakwell, 96 were returned (48 per cent) and only 39 of these were fully completed (19.5 per cent of the total sent), 39 were not completed and 18 were not completed but were returned with some appended information. Of the 39 respondents who returned uncompleted questionnaires, 18 claimed that they did not have enough time to do the questionnaire or were suffering under too heavy a workload. Seven said that the information required in the questionnaire was not available.

Breakwell found that there was a wide range of definitions of counselling among her respondents, but only clinical psychologists were expected to have qualifications in counselling before they were appointed. Other staff had a counselling element identified in their role and some training, usually brief and voluntary, was provided for them. Only 31 per cent of the 39 DHAs' representatives who completed the questionnaire could identify a budget for training in counselling. With such a low response rate any conclusions drawn from Breakwell's national survey must be treated cautiously and cannot be generalized.

In 1990 CMS was reorganized and a new constitution devised. The Executive remained concerned about how to best represent the diversity of its membership and fulfil its wide remit. A major influence in 1990 was the new contract for GPs. A working party was formed with the Royal College of General Practitioners to produce a clinical information folder for GPs on counselling in general practice, and the CMS guides on counselling in general practice were updated after funding was awarded by the Wellcome Foundation. Given the diversity of its membership it is appropriate that work was increasingly undertaken by subcommittees of the Division. There was a shift in emphasis to subgroups with two newly formed groups for Hospital Settings and Training. The Training subgroup was intended to be self-financing and took on the role of a working group rather than an advisory panel. The main achievements and progress continued to be in the Subcommittee on Counselling in General Practice which succeeded in achieving one of its major aims. A multi-agency working group was set up to formulate and agree national guidelines on counselling in general practice with representatives from CMS, BAC, British Psychological Society, Royal College of General Practitioners, Family Health Services Authority, Department of Health and Relate. These guidelines were launched at the House of Commons in May 1993. It is intended that all FHSAs and general practices in England and Wales will eventually receive a copy. An updated second edition of the guidelines will include an additional section to cover the placement of trainee counsellors in general practice.

There has been no national evaluation of counselling provision outside the primary care sector since Breakwell's 1987 survey. The rapid growth in membership of the CMS Division since 1990 gives some indication of the national picture of the development of counselling in medical settings. Following the successful launch of the general practice guidelines, emphasis has shifted within the Division towards meeting the needs of counsellors in hospital settings.

The CMS SubCommittee on Counselling in Hospital Settings is faced with a towering remit to raise the profile of counselling in hospital settings. This includes the provision of information and guidelines on the employment of counsellors in hospitals, their training in counselling and counselling skills, liaison, support and pay, and the collation of information and empirical research about counselling in hospital settings. Many staff in hospitals use the *Guidelines for the Employment of Counsellors in General Practice* (BAC 1993b) while they await publication of their own in 1995.

By September 1994 membership of the CMS Division within BAC had increased to 1097 individuals and 23 organizations; it is still the fastest growing division. The Executive Committee's aim is to liaise with other national organizations within this field in order to be able to respond more proactively to the stated needs of members and to promote and maintain professional standards of counselling in medical settings nationwide. Its intention is to offer a consultancy service to staff in institutions, health authorities and hospital trusts who are planning to implement counselling provision and a troubleshooting service for those who are experiencing difficulties within existing provision. New subcommittees are planned to coordinate developments in specialist training for counsellors in medical settings and in research and evaluation.

COUNSELLING IN GENERAL PRACTICE

The radical health care reforms following the new GP contract (1990) have accelerated the steady growth of counselling in primary health care that took place in the preceding decade. The *Guidelines for the Employment of Counsellors in General Practice* (BAC 1993b) which are being widely circulated to general practices in England and Wales, outline the role of the counsellor and give clear recommendations on training, job description, working as a member of the PHC Team, funding and employment status and insurance. The production of these guidelines was supported by the Counselling in Primary Care Trust which was established in 1991, sponsored by the Artemis Trust. The Counselling in Primary Care Trust is an important and proactive organization, committed to the establishment of a competent professional counselling service in primary health care. Its work includes the support, including funding, of local groups of general practitioners and counsellors, sponsorship of the development of a postgraduate Diploma at Masters level in Counselling in Primary Care, the promotion of conferences, symposia and workshops, sponsorship and commissioning of research into primary health care counselling, and the establishment of a research, citation and abstract database with free, open access. The Trust is also co-operating in the development of a more rigorous classification of the competencies involved in counselling which is being undertaken by the National Council for Vocational Qualifications (see p. 54).

The present position of counsellors within general practice shares some similarities with other occupational groups in health care. As new occupational identities emerge there are often initial difficulties in communication. Many of the current questions about the role of counsellors have previously been asked of doctors, nurses, health visitors and social workers – indeed of all of the allied and complementary practitioners working in general practice.

In June 1993 the funding system for health promotion clinics came to an end. Although this meant that some counsellors lost their jobs, it did focus attention more clearly on the central issues and priorities of what it meant to employ a counsellor within general practice. Those FHSAs which had funded counselling in general practice from the practice staff reimbursement scheme were not affected by the change.

Recognizing that primary care is usually the first point of contact for people seeking help with their emotional problems, Derbyshire FHSA implemented a counselling in general practice scheme in 1992. The late Viv Ball, former Chair of CMS' Counselling in General Practice Sub-Group, acted as a catalyst in this Authority, bringing her expertise, experience and conceptual understanding to this new initiative. Derbyshire FHSA supported its scheme by reimbursing the cost of the counsellor to the practice. This has ultimately led to a more stable service, shielded from the sudden shifts in short-term priority funding. By 1994 one-third of all practices in Derbyshire offered a counselling service. The scheme models the principles of good practice in counselling. To be eligible for employment counsellors have to fulfil certain criteria: they must be accredited by the BAC or its equivalent; have experience of working in primary care; have completed a formal programme of theoretical study; and have considerable experience of supervised practice. The scheme is well co-ordinated by a counselling and mental health adviser; training is a priority and supervision time costs are included in counsellors' contractual hours (Fitzgerald 1994). Derbyshire FHSA's *Guidelines for the Employment of Counsellors in Primary Care* (1994) includes detailed information on the role of the counsellor, contractual obligations, supervision, training and accreditation requirements, and professional liability insurance.

The growth and development of counselling in general practice reflects to a great extent the resources allocated to it. Fundholding practices and proactive FHSAs which are willing to implement, co-ordinate and fund the service become involved in producing guidelines, promoting training and research and including counsellors in their advisory groups. Some FHSAs are investigating the provision of counselling services but have no clear strategy for supporting the demand; others have not yet begun to include it within their strategic planning. The question of whether counselling in primary care should be allowed to develop through organic growth or be directed by NHS Management Executive policy mirrors the current diversity of and dilemmas about provision within FHSAs.

This brief historical overview has shown a continuous trend towards delegation of care in medical settings in which initial resistance is followed by incorporation; an increase in training and new qualifications with the medical network extending to incorporate the new specialist. This is the current position of counselling in medical settings. A key element in a quality service is appropriateness – the match between the assessment of patients' needs and provision. Who determines what is appropriate for whom? Features such as availability, accessibility, amenities, attitudes and responsiveness of staff are difficult to assess given both the subjectivity involved and the range of personal criteria for satisfaction. However, these factors are significant and need to balance quantitative measures such as numbers of re-admissions, referrals, repeat prescriptions and efficient budgeting, although research into the effectiveness and desirability of counselling services has also to somehow fit into this overall framework of monitoring and evaluation. This will be discussed in more depth in Chapter 4 but before that we will look more closely at the context of counselling in medical settings in Chapter 2.

· TWO ·

Counselling in medical settings

The territory of medical settings is vast and, like shifting sands, always on the move. It is impossible to do justice to the complexity, or to the way that different professional and lay groups and individuals perceive the overall landscape and their own particular part of it.

The medical world can be likened to a tribal village society. The ubiquitous visitor from Mars might discover a culture with a rich recorded history in addition to its folklore which has a complex system of values and beliefs and an established educational system rooted in science but also responsive to sponsorship and patronage by the elders and others who offer funds for research. Outsiders are excluded. There are strange rituals and ceremonial dress, peculiar rites of passage, apprenticeships and initiation tests, oaths of fealty and loyalty, both formal and informal codes of behaviour and rules of punishment and excommunication.

Newcomers – and counselling in medical settings is a newcomer – are often regarded with suspicion and hostility. Acceptance and incorporation into village life can take more than one generation. Until then the newcomers must adapt to the life of the village, grateful for the contact made by those who are interested and alert to the potential benefits of change. Alternatively they may become an alternative underground movement, like the tiny Borrowers (Mary Norton 1958) living behind the skirting boards of the big house, constantly under threat, watchful but also hugely resourceful, converting the scraps left behind by the big people into their own resources. Or the alternative underground movement might be much more abrasive, subversive and assertive in its demands for a piece of the action; setting up structures of its own, raising finance and recruiting grass roots support to confront the village elders and demand equal opportunities.

There are problems in defining the extent and nature of counselling in medical settings because the provision of counselling is so diverse, as is the context itself. As a result it is difficult to accurately evaluate current provision and therefore difficult to reach generalized conclusions. Counselling across all medical settings is at present essentially idiosyncratic in nature, lacking clear form and structures. So, although it is a phenomena that is growing, it is difficult to determine its pattern and shape.

There is now a growing amount of research into counselling in medical settings (see Chapter 4). What follows offers a global view of this work together with a more detailed examination of one of the major surveys, but the emphasis here will be on what practitioners and their patients/clients have to say about their experience of counselling in their own particular contexts.

In Chapter 1 we recognized the confusion and dilemma about where counselling fits into medical settings. Abel-Smith *et al.* (1989) point out that it is important to distinguish between the specific place in which counselling occurs and settings where a medical ethos reigns, i.e. the primary expectation is that a prescribed solution will be found for medical problems, with varying recognition being given to the interaction between physical, psychological and emotional issues.

Confusion is further compounded by the diversity in the nature and roles of the counsellors and their working arenas. Counsellors and other professional groups who view counselling as a significant area of their work are to be found working individually and in teams in primary health care, community health centres, specialist clinics, hospitals and therapeutic communities. The effects of the diversity of these settings are further intensified by the range of different counselling philosophies, expectations, values, beliefs and theoretical underpinnings and practice amongst the other members of the team.

Diversity can have its advantages. At best it offers a range of choice that in ideal form is matched to client need. However, although it is valuable to have a wide range of services, they need to work in a complementary (Pietroni 1993) and co-operative way to be effective. Conflicting or different aims are not effective. Then the issues of dominance, ownership and territorial rights (the term 'my patients' is often heard) can lead to competition and rivalrous spoiling of other team members' work. The following example demonstrates how patients seeing counsellors can be undermined by unhelpful and inappropriate responses from other professionals. When Dora told the consultant that she was seeing a counsellor after her hysterectomy, the patronizing tone of his reply 'if it helps you to talk dear. . .' left her in no doubt as to his feelings on the value of counselling. She, on the other hand, had no doubts and had set up a ring of support which included not only her family and friends and her counsellor but also involvement in a self-help group. In this instance Dora was sufficiently confident to judge for herself what was helpful to her. Other patients in similar situations, who are often distressed and vulnerable, may not be able to cope so assertively with unhelpful comments.

CONFUSED ABOUT WHAT COUNSELLORS DO?

Inevitably such confusions lead to genuine anxieties as well as conservative resistance. Another confusion may arise over the distinction between counselling skills and counselling. Hopefully, most, if not all, of the staff working in medical settings will be aware of the need to listen attentively, respond appropriately and give feedback when necessary, in a way that takes account of the individual's needs. These are all necessary for effective interpersonal relationships but do not, in themselves, constitute counselling. In this sense counselling skills are widespread, but counselling as such is a different modality requiring considerably more training and operating at a different and greater depth. Whereas most people can be trained to use counselling skills as part of a wider job, fewer are able to work as counsellors.

Counselling in this context is taken to be in line with BAC's definition:

> The overall aim of counselling is to provide an opportunity for the client to work towards living in a more satisfying and resourceful way. The term 'counselling' includes work with individuals, pairs or groups of people often, but not always, referred to as 'clients'. The objectives of particular counselling relationships will vary according to the client's needs. Counselling may be concerned with developmental issues, addressing and resolving specific problems, making decisions, coping with crisis, developing personal insight and knowledge, working through feelings of inner conflict or improving relationships with others. The counsellor's role is to facilitate the client's work in ways which respect the client's values, personal resources and capacity for self-determination.

Only when both the user and the recipient explicitly agree to enter into a counselling relationship does it become counselling rather than the use of 'counselling skills'. It is not possible to make a generally accepted distinction between counselling and psychotherapy. There are well-founded traditions which use the terms interchangeably and others which distinguish them. Regardless of the theoretical approaches preferred by individual counsellors, there are ethical issues which are common to all counselling situations.

(BAC 1993a)

In its *Code of Ethics and Practice for Counselling Skills* BAC states:

The term 'counselling skills' does not have a single definition which is universally accepted. For the purpose of this code, 'counselling skills' are distinguished from 'listening skills' and from 'counselling'. Although the distinction is not always a clear one, because the term 'counselling skills' contains elements of these other two activities, it has its own place in the continuum between them. What distinguishes the use of counselling skills from these other two activities are the intentions of the user, which is to enhance the performance of their functional role, as line manager, nurse, tutor, social worker, personnel officer, voluntary worker, etc., the recipient will, in turn, perceive them in that role.

(BAC 1989)

If you are not sure about whether you are a counsellor or use counselling skills as an integral aspect of your role, ask yourself these questions from BAC to help clarify your status:

1 Are you using counselling to enhance your communication with someone but without taking on the role of their counsellor?
2 Does the recipient perceive you as acting within your professional/caring role (which is NOT that of being their counsellor)?

i   If the answer is YES to both these questions, you are using counselling skills in your functional role.
ii If the answer is NO to both, you are counselling and should look to the *Code of Ethics and Practice for Counsellors* for guidance.
iii If the answer is YES to one and NO to the other, you have a conflict of expectations and should resolve it.

(BAC 1989)

Syme (1993) identifies 143 theoretical approaches to counselling found in the BAC's *Counselling and Psychotherapy Resources Directory* of

which 20 were included in its membership survey (1993). It is
likely that many counsellors and therapists working in medical
settings fit into the broad bands of psychodynamic, humanistic and
cognitive/behavioural approaches. In the following case studies three
practising counsellors Su, Gilbert and Connor, describe how these
theoretical approaches inform their practice. For those readers wishing to know more about these and other approaches, Dryden (1984)
has produced a comprehensive view of individual therapies.

SU – A PSYCHODYNAMIC COUNSELLOR IN
GENERAL PRACTICE

I work for 12 hours a week as a counsellor in a general practice. I
have two hours supervision per month which is paid for by my
employers, but I am not paid for the time. My post was funded
from the 70 per cent ancillary funding arrangements until 1993,
when the FHSA in my area took over existing services. I am a
qualified counsellor, having completed a three-year part-time university programme in psychodynamic counselling. The FHSA guidelines in my area stipulate that counsellors in general practice should
be accredited by BAC or Relate. The GPs retain clinical responsibility for all of my clients (actually, I call them patients which I suppose reflects my alliance with the doctors and nursing staff). They
make referrals to me, there is no provision for self-referral. During
my time at the practice referrals have become more appropriate
because there's more opportunity for feedback on whether someone
is suitable for counselling. I see people for various lengths of time,
the average contact being 15 sessions, but I do have autonomy to
extend or renegotiate contracts according to individual needs.

My contact with the GPs and other staff is mostly informal and
ad hoc. I have an occasional meeting with the practice's health visitor but my main contacts are with the general practitioners, in
particular when they ask for feedback on someone's progress. My
boundary of confidentiality includes keeping notes, recording starting and ending dates and comments about attendance. I find that
I can maintain confidentiality regarding the content of counselling
sessions and still co-operate with the practice's protocol on record
keeping. I don't have a medical training but I don't think that this
is a disadvantage. When I need information about medication or
physical features of illness I ask one of the general practitioners. I
think this is preferable to having a mental set which might medicalize

a presenting issue. However, I also think that my role demands more than basic counselling skills. My current training includes issues like assessment of a person's suitability for counselling. There needs to be real collaboration between me and all other staff about the appropriateness of referrals to me and referrals from me out to the local psychological, psychiatric and psychotherapy units. I also see my role as being supportive to the doctors when they become upset and anxious because there is nothing they can do.

My training has mainly been psychodynamic, that's the approach I use for long-term work, though my range extends to basically supporting people through difficult periods in their lives, when I don't say very much at all. Words are not the only means of communication, they fail us often when we need them most. The deepest human experiences always seem to defy the capacity of language to describe them. However, the meaning that the client makes out of our dialogue is central so I would call it a talking treatment. The main influences on my work are from the Object Relations School, Klein, Fairbairn, Winnicott, Balint. My broad definition of object relations would include the understanding that people live simultaneously in an external world and in an internal world with varying degrees of awareness and adaptation. The *objects* in object relations theory can be real external people, things or conditions such as illness and they can also be experienced as internal images. Externally or internally, it is the way that a person's self becomes an essential partner in relationships with itself and others that is the cornerstone of object relations theories. So, my work with people takes very much into account how they relate to themselves and to me during our sessions as well as how they describe other relationships in their lives. This is what is meant by the *transference*, the way that thoughts, feelings and expectations, both recent and ancient, are transferred from the person's experience of the past into the here and now with me. Object relations theories assumes that behaviour in the counselling relationship represents experiences brought forward from other, often very early, object relations when the person behaves as if the counsellor were his or her mother/ father/brother/sister.

The client and I talk about his/her thoughts and feelings. Some of these thoughts and feelings are implicit in the words that are used, or the way they are said, but cannot be made explicit if, for good defensive reasons, the client has no insight into them or permission to hold them. As well as listening to what the client says I listen for the way that s/he censors or prohibits the expression of certain ideas and feelings. It's like prohibition in America – illicit arrangements have to be made, secret venues and 'speak-easies' arranged – enabling the client to express forbidden thoughts through slips of the tongue, jokes, puns, and sometimes in physical symptoms. Sometimes people don't have a repertoire of language to express their hurt or angry feelings or they may be too frightened to say what they feel. If clients cannot describe their feelings, they sometimes act them out, so, for example, someone might feel very tense and literally feel it with stiffness in the body. Counselling is about working together on an alternative way of expressing the feelings and to look at some of the possible causes. If clients do not use an 'as if' kind of language, I might introduce them to this way of thinking by using it myself.

By helping the person to make connections between what is happening in the counselling relationship and those earlier experiences it becomes possible for him or her to gain more insight and understanding of the 'as if' experiences. Permission for the client to entertain an idea is fostered if I am able to understand and tolerate his or her thoughts and feelings. Then the client can begin to be able to talk about these experiences with me rather than perpetually re-enact them. For example, Ken, whom I saw weekly for 12 sessions, is a middle-aged man, successful in his work, with a stable marriage and home life, but he kept visiting the doctor complaining of severe pains across his chest and upper arms for which no physical cause could be found. Soon after I had started working with Ken he told me, almost incidentally, about the death of his eldest child. I didn't realize for a while that he was talking about a child who had died almost 30 years ago.

I am alert to the ways that people's past experiences roll up behind them and are re-experienced, re-enacted even, in the present, but I was surprised by how recent Ken's story sounded. Ken thought it was odd that I encouraged him to talk about his feelings and to reflect on what had happened in the past. He thought I would want him to describe his physical pains. He didn't really have a repertoire of language to describe his feelings. Over the next few weeks it became clearer that ever since childhood the only way that Ken could express his hurt feelings was to actually feel the hurt of pain in his body. He would often preface a sentence with solicitous remarks about my feelings or 'I'm sure you don't want to hear all this.' When it became possible for Ken to say how hurt he felt he began to get some relief from the pain and eventually made the connection himself after he said he felt broken-hearted when his child had died but couldn't tell his family because he had to be the strong one.

GILBERT – A PERSON-CENTRED COUNSELLOR WORKING IN A UNIVERSITY HEALTH CENTRE

I work primarily in a person-centred way. I use Carl Rogers' philosophy and model of counselling to underpin my work, and to structure the way I work with clients. It has a very strong bias towards people having a positive self-direction, towards self-actualizing, given the right environment. By self-actualizing I mean really to truly be oneself, to become more genuine, so that behaviour and feelings are more in line with conscious thoughts.

The whole approach is centred around present time, around being in the present, not looking backwards into causes, or forwards into problem management, it stays very much in the moment. In counselling sessions when clients experience something totally new I would help them to stay in that moment, in the present. The experience may come from the past but the emphasis is placed on how the person feels about it and relates right now. Rogers accepted and was aware of unconscious and transference issues, but in the person-centred model of counselling they're not made the primary focus, they're just a part of the present time relationship with the client. As the unconscious becomes more conscious, there's a greater self-awareness and understanding.

The person-centred counselling model came out of Rogers' original non-directive model which is a good place to start because the techniques and ideas that started there are still used by client or person-centred counsellors nowadays. For example, a counsellor might recognize or interpret the feeling that the client is expressing directly, or by their general demeanor, or specific behaviour, or from earlier statements. Crucially, a non-directive counsellor would not try to direct the content of the dialogue. However, Rogers recognized that just using techniques was not enough and in developing client-centred therapy he stressed the importance of the quality of the relationship between the client and the counsellor. He came up with three main elements or core conditions of the counsellor's behaviour or attitude which were crucial to the quality of the relationship. The first one is that counsellors need to be genuine and aware of their inner feelings. They may choose not to express them, but at times, I guess probably more so than some in other models of counselling, they may well choose to express their feelings to their clients if they felt that it was appropriate. There's often more self-disclosure than in other models of counselling. For me it's about getting an intuitive sense of what is appropriate for me to share with a client. I tend to err on the cautious side. The important thing is that there is congruence between what I feel and how I am with the client.

Second, Rogers said that it was crucial for the counsellor to be acceptant of the client. This is about valuing the client and prizing him or her. The client and the counsellor have a warm relationship, that is something that is generally recognized to be prevalent in a person-centred counselling relationship. Rogers' third core condition is empathy. The counsellor needs to be empathic towards clients, a deep, sensitive understanding which involves entering their private worlds, so that the counsellor is really in there struggling alongside them with their understanding of themselves. This co-exists along-side an acceptance of the client as a separate person. Being em-pathic does not mean becoming totally submerged, it means having the strength to remain separate while being with the client in his or her own world.

I was trained at Bristol University where they put a very strong emphasis on humanistic approaches to counselling, broader than just the Carl Rogers person-centred model. I spent five years in training doing various courses but the most significant was the Diploma in Counselling which I did part-time for two years. It was an eclectic course that helped me to integrate different models of counselling within a very holding structure. My training very much mirrored the way I work now. I guess the only other thing that I will mention is that, particularly in the late stages of his life, Carl Rogers started emphasizing spirituality as another dimension. I think that for me is also a natural extension of the person-centred way of working.

My work with Issie shows the theory in practice. I have been seeing her for about a year now. She has chosen to come to this university, only a short distance from where she lives with her parents. In the first year of her course Issie was coping with sepa-ration from her parents relatively well, although she was having some panic attacks and had been prescribed minor tranquillizers here at the health centre. In the second year of the course she started becoming extremely uncomfortable about being separated from her parents and came to see me at the counselling service. Issie was very anxious in the sessions. I recognized that and ac-cepted that anxiety as a part of her without judging it. Slowly Issie started to accept her own behaviour and feelings, for example, about having to go home in the middle of the week to stay overnight with her parents, as being part of what she needed at that point in her life. Issie began to be able to accept that anxious part of herself and instead of giving herself a really hard time about it (she was very good at beating herself up) she was able to acknowledge that that was her stage of development at the moment. Instead of setting herself goals like 'I must, I ought, I should, I have got to stay here at the university for a whole week and not go back and see my parents other than at the weekends' and failing, she began to accept that it was OK for her to go home if she had to. She started dropping some of the goals which were unrealistic for her to achieve and started becoming more congruent, her behaviour started to match the way she actually felt about the situation. Linked in with all that, throughout the relationship, I've tried to be as empathic with Issie's situation as possible and to enter into her private world to try and explore and understand the kind of feelings which have been going on for her, in order to understand her difficulty in separating. Now this helps to illustrate the process as well because Issie's experience fits the directions in therapy that Rogers talks about. She began to experience her potential self in the sessions so that instead of just being trapped in her patterned way of thinking she started saying, 'I don't have to be like this.' Issie started to feel the full experience of a relationship in counselling in which she was unconditionally accepted. The next stage was a liking of herself, and she actually came to accept herself, whether or not she was having to return home. Issie didn't actually like the fact that she had to go home but she ended up accepting it. She's discovered that the core of her personality is positive rather than clinging to the doubts around what was inside her as a person. In our sessions Issie can now recognize for herself the feelings and experiences that are going on inside her. She can actually be in the moment rather than describe her thoughts and feelings in the third person. The irony of all of this is that while she was trying to create this goal for herself, pushing herself to stay at the university for a whole week without seeing her parents, she could not achieve it. When she dropped it as a goal and just allowed herself to do what she needed to she found it easier and was able to stay at university for the whole of last term.

Issie was able to talk through her own feelings about taking drugs and decided that she did not want to take the tablets but she knew that that option was there as a backup. I acknowledge as a person-centred counsellor that if somebody feels as though they have to take prescribed drugs because their anxiety is so great, they can play a role for that person at that time. That might be their need. It's very necessary for me to know how different drugs may be affecting particular clients and the sort of counselling work they may be capable of doing. I have to say that I find communications about this weak. It is something on which I would like to see psychiatrists place a greater emphasis. It's a tricky one because of boundaries and confidentiality but often clients who are also seeing psychiatrists want that kind of increased holding; a lot of them do actually want that sort of link.

The referrals from the doctors vary. Some are not appropriate in that the client obviously does not want to come to the counselling service and is only there because the doctors recommended it. So a number of referrals don't get past the first session. It is important for me to establish whether that person actually wants to be in a counselling relationship. On many occasions though, clients do come and want to use the relationship effectively and they probably would not have come if they had not been referred. Students can self-refer too.

The issues of confidentiality do need careful attention. Other staff sometimes want to know how well students are doing in counselling. I do take the opportunity on those occasions to explain about boundaries around counselling and their importance. It's a chance to explain something of the process of counselling without talking about that particular client. Sometimes I find myself being a counsellor for other carers, giving a background support to them when they are working with students. That goes for people within the wider institution as well as within this team, the tutors and other members of staff.

CONNOR – A COGNITIVE BEHAVIOURAL COUNSELLOR WORKING IN A SPECIALIST SUBSTANCE MISUSE UNIT

A couple of years ago I looked at the Rogerian approach and felt that it fitted in with a generic community psychiatric nurse's (CPN) approach because it is very much client-centred. When you are entering peoples' own homes, you've got to take their world into account. I think too many people hide behind the desk in the office and expect people to come to them. Then I did further training in Sheffield. I did a nine-month cultural behavioural project based on a Rogerian approach. That was the background to my being drawn towards a cognitive behavioural aspect which fitted in with what I was already doing and actually gave it more structure.

While I was on the course I was introduced to cognitive theorists like Beck and Ellis. The thing I really picked up on, and use a lot, is looking at people's automatic thoughts when faced with certain situations, how that makes them feel and how that affects the way they live their lives. I believe in educating clients about what is going on so that they can really understand how to change. When I started working as a CPN again it really changed my work and made it a lot more structured. I was seeing clients for less time and doing far more with them in the time I was spending with them and I felt far more satisfied with the sort of work I was doing. I felt I was actually getting somewhere and I knew why I had been successful with this person and not with that one, whereas before I was a bit unsure. I think that the course was also a good education for me. It helped me to understand more about anxiety and the ins and outs of depressions that I should have learned about before I became a CPN. It's helped me to understand what people are going through and to stop making classic mistakes like not saying, 'Ah, don't worry about anxiety, it's not going to kill you.' It does, it does kill people. I learned good protocols. For example, if somebody comes to me with anxiety, I always make sure they have been checked out for physical causes first, whereas before I did not necessarily do that. I was also able to pass on information to my colleagues who had not done the course. The GPs loved it. They would ring and refer somebody and I would say, 'Hang on, before they're referred, have you done this, that and the other,' and they would ask 'why?' and I would reply, 'Well, it could be this, that or the other' and they would say, 'Oh I didn't think about that, I'll check it out' and they would do all the tests and send the information through to me which was good. I also learnt about post-traumatic stress disorders and things like that – topical stuff at the time, which I recognized in one or two of the clients I'd already been seeing. Because we were only allowed to take three clients on at any one time when we were doing the course it allowed me to work in-depth with them in an ideal sort of setting.

I found the course excellent, it's the best thing that I think has happened to me as far as my professional training is concerned. It's that important. As far as I'm concerned it was my personal development towards offering what I think is a good service. What happened after a while was that I had changed too much to actually carry on working where I was. I had been there for four years and I felt that I was being held back. Then this job came up in a specialist unit working with substance misuse. I'd already read about using a cognitive behavioural approach with substance misuse and it sounded quite exciting so I did a bit more reading and also went to meet the consultant and talk to him about the other people who were involved. I thought, 'Yes, this is what I want to do.' It's very structured and very clear about the counselling role and it was also very clear that bringing a cognitive behavioural background was what they wanted. I began looking at the sort of models that were being used within substance misuse.

One that seemed to be universally used was a trans-theoretical model so it actually fitted in with whatever approach was being used. The Prochaska and Di Clementi model was developed around helping smokers to stop smoking. It's a circular staged model which starts off with a pre-contemplation stage, moves on to a contemplation stage and then on to an action stage and finally on to the maintenance stage. You can use whatever approach you want to move people around it and the cognitive behavioural approach fits in very nicely. People move on very quickly and it offers a quick intervention. If they relapse, and substance misuse is a chronic relapsing condition, they move back into the pre-contemplation stage and repeat the cycle. So the model is really something that applies to everyone that we see because it gives a way of identifying at which stage somebody is. Are they in pre-contemplation, are they contemplating change, are they actually trying to change, are they struggling with maintaining change or are they about to re-lapse? It was OK then to go back to the people that I had read like Beck or Ellis and use some of their approaches with people with substance misuse problems. I found that I could use Beck's model of depression, which looks at how a critical incident might then activate negative thoughts, automatic negative thoughts with re-lapse, seeing how people deal with stress. They automatically go and have a drink, which sets off a lot of negative thinking about whether they are able to cope. We teach people to try and learn more positive ways of thinking or less demanding ways of dealing with stress. We focus on what may set off the substance misuse, and if that works well, we move from contemplative mode to actually changing, getting them to confront and challenge the situation. We get people to explain things to us. We help them engage their own thinking and help them to challenge themselves by challenging them. I find that really quite powerful and they find it powerful too, it gives them something to hang on to.

We have set up a relapse prevention group which is very struc-tured, based around education, lasting over six sessions, each session having a different theme, and it is working well in spite of common opinion that group work is not suitable for substance misusers. I'm a good salesman with what I do because that's part of it, showing people that I believe in what I do. We hold on to people when normally they wouldn't stay with a service like ours. Nationally there's about a 40 per cent drop out rate, we've got a 15 per cent drop out rate and most people go through the full course. I believe our high retention rate is due to our attitude towards people who have normally been written off by others. I try to show them that they are not just a diagnosis or a condition to be treated. We don't use the term alcoholic, we use the term *a person with alcohol problems*. We don't use the term substance abuse, we use the term *substance misuse* because abuse has its own connotations, though I do belong to an organization called the Association of Nurses in Substance Abuse.

One of my clients was in his late thirties, divorced with two children, a guy with a good trade, a plumber, who worked on his own, very successful, found the stress at work very hard. About 15 years ago he began using alcohol as a way of coping and relaxing and switching off, but this increased and he started to drink at work. This started to have an effect on his marriage, but he believed that he did not have a problem and so it continued. Eventually his marriage split up, he lost contact with his son, and fell out with his parents because they could see that he had a problem with it as well, but he remained adamant that he was in control. He rented a caravan and just worked to fund his alcohol. He set up a network where he could always get a drink, whatever the time of day. He was in debt all the time, and he became very angry, angry with the world in general, feeling that it had given him a bad deal. Gradually his health was deteriorating. We're talking about a 38-year-old man who is starting to show signs of serious liver damage, not necessarily irreversible but getting to the point where he was at risk of causing himself a lot of permanent damage. He started to steal, even, on one occasion in front of his small son. He was now stealing and lying and getting argumentative; he'd stopped caring about himself, his appearance and just lived for the next drink. By chance he ended up getting admitted to Accident and Emergency through an alcohol overdose and was moved over to the psychiatric unit. He spent a couple of days in there before we were contacted. We recognized that if we let go of this guy he would go straight back out and start drinking again. I got him to look at his life, look at what was really going on and ask him whether that was what he really wanted. He had not had a drink for over a week and was surviving without alcohol. I thought that he wouldn't do very well because he wasn't ready and I wasn't sure if I could move him on to actually being ready. I decided to try and get him into a Social Services rehabilitation unit where I could maintain contact with him. He could be independent but there was 24-hour cover. He had been through a detoxification and come out the other side – he'd now spent a week without any medication or a drink and he started to present anxiety problems about not being able to cope with every-day things without drinking. There was also a lot of grieving going on as he began to face the loss of the life he had once had.

I used cognitive behavioural therapy to teach him about negative thinking and about how that affected the way he felt and behaved. He took that on board very, very quickly and found it really useful because it gave him a way of understanding what was going on. It also empowered him because it gave him the ability to challenge his own negative thinking so he didn't need me around all the time. I also taught him relaxation and diversional techniques. He then moved into the relapse prevention group. He was actually in the first one that we ran. It was cognitive-based, structured over a six-week period and people turned up one afternoon a week. It was a small group with six to eight people but they spent quite a bit of time with each other and they were all in a similar position although they all had their own individual problems. We looked at issues such as coping with anxiety and depression, recognizing it, what you can do about it, lifestyle changes, filling time, high-risk situations in the past that have caused relapse, and generally chal-lenging the past behaviour against what could happen now if they really wanted it. I was absolutely amazed that we had a 100 per cent retention rate for the six weeks. My client moved from being a quite withdrawn, suspicious sort of person to being quite a vocal and respected member of the group.

When that started to happen he began to realize that he had a lot of hidden skills in that he was good at talking to people, he had something to offer and off his own back he actually went and got himself a voluntary job at a local nursing home. They were so impressed with him that they wanted to take him on as a paid worker, but at the same time he'd also got himself a voluntary job working with people with learning disabilities at Social Services. They were so impressed with him that they did offer him a full-time job and that is what he is doing now, he's now left the rehabilitation unit, he's got himself a place to live, he sees his son every weekend, he is talking to his wife, his parents really respect him and he's not ever relapsed – although he has been very close. What he has done, and this is something cognitive/behavioural work enables, is to learn to recognize the early signs and what to do about them. He is now helping us to set up a follow-up to the groups that we run where the groups can continue to meet and offer each other support. He'd been written off, he'd been called an alcoholic, a down and out, a vagrant because that was how he was living, but underneath it all he was very skilled, a very worthwhile person with a lot to offer.

COUNSELLING IN PRIMARY HEALTH CARE TEAMS

In this section we look at provision in primary health care settings. This is the area where the greatest progress has been made towards clarifying provision and practice in counselling, in particular with the production of *Guidelines for the Employment of Counsellors in General Practice* (BAC 1993). The developments in counselling provision in PHC are not necessarily matched by a corresponding increase in understanding what counsellors do or what makes counselling effective. Nor is the provision developing in a coherent and systematic way in all areas throughout Britain. Perhaps confusion is inevitable and the only possible response when there is little agreement nationally about the nature and delivery of counselling and a wide array of disparate provision is on offer. There is a clear need for research to establish what separates effective counselling from the wide range of services currently available in order for training to be focused accordingly (Tyrer, Higgs and Strathdee 1993).

Glenys Parry from the Department of Health opened the December 1993 conference on 'Counselling and Primary Mental Health Care: Promoting Good Practice' by saying that general practitioners and FHSAs were buying counselling but it was not always clear what it was they were getting for their money. The term *counselling* is being used to cover almost any psychological work in primary care, from those using counselling skills to specialist focused psychotherapy interventions. There have been a number of descriptive local surveys which suggest that counselling services are valued by GPs and patients and are of particular value for those who lack social support. However, there is a dearth of evidence for the effectiveness of counselling in improving mental health. It tends to be an isolated provision, sitting somewhat uneasily in a no-man's-land between primary and secondary health care. The Department of Health's view is that vision and collaboration are needed to overcome a lack of coordination of mental health care and to foster the growth of provision for the treatment of mental health problems in primary care settings. The concern is that any growth in provision should lead to safe and effective practice, the early detection of depression and anxiety, and accessible, local and friendly services that are well coordinated with secondary care and will improve the counselling skills of all practice staff. For this to happen there needs to be systematic monitoring and evaluation of provision and dissemination of information. This may require central leadership or it could develop from pluralism and organic growth. The expansion in counselling provision in primary health care could well be described as pluralistic and organic. This is a more generous description to the alternative interpretation that it is confused and geographically patchy.

Counselling in general practice, is a more widely researched and documented area of counselling in medical settings, and these developments are well summarized in Corney and Jenkins (1993), Sheldon (1992) and information available from the Counselling in Primary Care Trust. Guides for general practitioners and counsellors in general practice have been issued by the Counselling in Medical Settings Division of BAC since 1985. As referred to in Chapter 1, a comprehensive set of guidelines for the employment of counsellors in general practices was published in 1993 following three years of consultation with key professionals in this field of work. This publication reflects the growing need for a lucid and coherent framework to match the growth in numbers of counsellors employed in this setting since 1990 and the changes in general practice.

There are a number of differently qualified staff who may describe themselves as counsellor in a general practice, with great variations in training, therapeutic orientation and casework mix. The range spans individuals with little or no training and experience offering a few hours of unsupervised counselling each week across a professional spectrum which includes doctors, nurses, social workers, occupational therapists, psychiatrists, psychotherapists and chartered psychologists. This has clear and concerning implications for evaluating a service (Corney 1990). The BAC's guidelines on employment focus on the need to attend to this variation in training and status and the need to clarify the role and function of the counsellor, particularly for fundholding practices in the light of changes in mental health services.

In their study of counselling as a distinct or separate service within general practice, Sibbald, Addington-Hall, Brenneman and Freeling (1993) conducted a major survey of counselling services in 1,180 general practices in England and Wales. Of the 82 per cent (1,542) who responded, a total of 875 doctors said that their practice provided a counselling service. However not all of these met the research criterion that there was a person on site, or within the practice, who:

offers formal sessions to patients in which patients are helped to define their problems and enabled to reach their own solutions. General practitioners and others provide counselling in the

ordinary course of their work, but we need to know about the
provision of counselling as a distinct or separate activity within
the practice.

(Sibbald *et al*. 1993:30)

Taking this definition of counselling as a separate, distinct service
the research found that there were 586 counsellors distributed among
484 of the 1,542 practices. There was a predominance of three types
of counsellor: community psychiatric nurses (187); practice counsellors (145); and clinical psychologists (95). In addition to differences in counselling provision according to the health region there
were various other factors which predicted the presence of a counsellor within a practice. Having four or more partners employed in
the practice was a major factor in deciding whether to employ community psychiatric nurses. Practices which employed staff who were
specifically designated *counsellor* were more likely to be training
practices and to provide stress clinics. Clinical psychologists were
also more likely to be employed in training practices and in practices with a list size of more than 10,500 patients. Only 197 of the
counsellors were trained in counselling. Even more alarmingly, the
qualifications of 85 of the counsellors were unknown to the general
practitioner – or at least to the person completing the questionnaire. Of the 667 doctors who did not have a counsellor, 413 said
that they would like to provide one, 85 were opposed to the idea,
144 were uncertain and 25 did not respond. The barriers to providing a counsellor were financial constraints (251); lack of space (136);
lack of time (81); staffing difficulties (72); low demand (29); doubt
about the value of counselling (15); and other reasons (52).

Sibbald *et al*. conclude that because of their focus on counselling
as a distinct and separate service their survey provided a conservative estimate of the true prevalence of counselling services. Even so,
the study confirmed a previously suspected rapid growth in such
services, suggesting that 31 per cent of all general practices had
counsellors with no other job in the practice with a further four-
fifths (80 per cent) of the general practitioners in their survey without a counsellor in the practice wishing to provide one.

The most likely setting for separate counselling provision was in
large practices and training practices. The practical implications of
generating more accommodation, funding and workload are linked
to larger practices and, as the researchers point out, training practices are expected to be at the leading edge of innovation. Provision
of financial incentives for stress clinics permitted the general practitioners to be reimbursed under their new contracts leading to an

expansion in the employment of counsellors but this was an unsatisfactory pragmatic alternative in the absence of a coherent funding policy. Funding arrangements via family health service authorities appeared inconsistent and variable though the researchers acknowledge that further research is needed to investigate these effects.

The counsellors in this survey undertook a wide variety of work, which reflected the doctors' perceptions of their competence. The community psychiatric nurses were seen to be appropriate for management of psychiatric illnesses including affective and psychotic disorders. Clinical psychologists tended to receive referrals for problems such as psycho-sexual difficulties, eating disorders, phobias and obsessive compulsive disorders which link with the behavioural therapies often associated with these professionals. Bereaved patients were most often seen by practice counsellors. Like Corney (1990), this research showed that all counsellors had referred to them a wide range of problems from patients experiencing family difficulties to psychiatric disorders, a challenge for the most experienced of counsellors and an indication of the need for an appropriate and discriminating referral policy and adequate training and supervision.

Annalee Curran describes how she uses Cognitive Analytic Therapy (CAT) with selected clients at the GP practice where she works as a practice counsellor (Curran and Higgs 1993). CAT was originated by Dr Anthony Ryle, drawing on cognitive and analytic theories, as a means of offering time limited therapy which also has the potential to work with a patient in some depth. The approach focuses on identifying underlying patterns of behaviour, thought and belief (called traps, dilemmas and snags) which are repeated to such an extent that people can become stuck in a cycle of dysfunctional behaviour which is spoiling their lives. The cognitive components of CAT include identifying these patterns; naming the core pain; reformulation of the patients' stories and of their patterns (written and diagrammatical), using their own words and images; and enlisting the patients' active involvement in homework tasks between sessions. The ending of therapy is marked by good-bye letters – summaries of progress and achievements and of how the patients will continue the work themselves – which are exchanged between patient and therapist. CAT is an integrative model which uses educative and problem-solving approaches while taking account of deep, hidden feelings. It encourages patients to get a clearer understanding of themselves and to make changes on a more cognitive level. It is also time limited and essentially an active approach, requiring considerable input from the patient and the therapist but not to the exclusion of the dynamic therapeutic relationship.

COUNSELLING IN SECONDARY HEALTH CARE

'Struck Off and Die' are Tony Gardner and Phil Hammond, an alternative comedy duo who qualified as doctors in 1987, met while working as house officers in Bristol and started writing and performing together in 1990. Tony is a qualified GP and is currently working full-time as a writer and actor. Phil is a lecturer in General Practice at Birmingham University. Their material is horribly realistic, drawn from their own experiences. One of their sketches revolves around the desperate need of a junior hospital doctor for a meal. So hungry is he, after missed opportunities throughout the day and night, that he agrees, like a young prince in a fairy story who is set the task of finding the correct answer to a riddle in order to win the hand of a princess, to complete four tasks set by the nursing staff, for the prize of a box of chocolates belonging to one of the patients. The four tasks include everyday experiences such as taking a blood sample and having to tell a patient bad news.

Of course, the junior fails because by the time he has dealt sensitively with the four tasks, all of the chocolates have been eaten. He is then shown the ropes by an old hand – this mentor shows our young doctor how to dump all four tasks back on to the nursing staff or the patients in less than a minute and so get to eat. Phil Hammond and Tony Gardner powerfully illustrate some very serious issues for doctors through their black comedy. They use their own excellent skills of communication to demonstrate that there is often an abyss between what is needed and what is available.

Secondary health care is more cosmopolitan, and consequently more difficult to categorize, than primary health care which tends to have a defined locality or neighbourhood. With greater involvement of specialist and different occupational groups, counselling has yet to emerge as a distinct form of treatment. The position in this context is roughly where counselling in primary health care was about 10–15 years ago. A working party coordinated by the Counselling in Medical Settings Division of BAC was established in 1994 to produce guidelines for the employment of counsellors in hospital settings. The contribution of volunteers and lay support is enormously important in supporting clinical medicine, often providing counselling services and telephone help lines to patients and their families who would not otherwise have any opportunity for contact (Tyndall 1993).

Counselling in secondary health care is probably the most patchy and varied of all provision in medical settings. We have no clear, overall picture of this provision. There have been no national surveys of provision in this context since Breakwell's 1987 survey. Many counsellors in secondary health care settings wear two hats. They are employed to work as counsellors in conjunction with a role linked to another occupational identity such as nursing or radiography which may take priority when there are staff shortages or a lack of resources. Doctors in hospitals are much more likely to be familiar with the practices of psychology, psychotherapy and psychiatry than with counselling as a discipline in its own right.

I will introduce you now to five students from a large medical school in the North-East of England. You will meet them again in the following chapters. I conducted a small survey with this group, two young women and three young men, to check out their understanding of counselling issues and to find out whether they had received any training or preparation for counselling. Asked what they understood counselling to mean, they replied:

Specific interviews or psychotherapy in which an expert on the subject (the counsellor) provides a client with desirable information (whether mechanisms of coping or just simple information). There can be 'passive' (just listening) or 'active' imparting of information.

Counselling refers to the interactive process by which the counsellor discusses a topic with a person and during which the counsellor may provide an explanation, provide relevant information, offer advice, and help the person to make a decision.

Counselling is a process whereby someone familiar with a topic or situation offers or gives advice to a person ignorant in respect to the situation. This may occur in a variety of settings whereby the information provided is purely factual, or more usually it is directed, in an attempt for the person to gain insight into a situation so that they may ultimately draw their own conclusions about the implications for themselves and others, so they may understand, accept or (if necessary) make informed decisions about the situation in question (e.g. genetic counselling).

Counselling – listening, offering advice and support to patient and family. Working with the person with difficulties to overcome difficulties (problems) so they can make an informed decision.

Counselling – therapeutic instruction given in order to help an individual or group in order to aid them in a particular situation.

These trainee doctors appear to construe counselling as being involved with giving advice and information. It is impossible to make any generalized assumptions from this small sample but the trainees' responses do match Breakwell's findings (see p. 131).

The inexperienced or naïve view of mental health care is that all staff are trained and competent in counselling or counselling skills; the reality is that psychiatric nurses and psychiatrists are as likely to follow a medical model of treatment as nurses and doctors in general hospitals. Psychiatrists are not required to be supervised in the way that most counsellors and psychotherapists would regard as crucial to their work and even in settings specifically concerned with mental health the provision of counselling cannot be taken for granted.

Contemporary medical training, it is claimed, (Seale and Pattison 1994) gives much more time and attention to the need to develop interpersonal and communication skills. Our medical students from the North-East gave the following replies to the question 'Have you observed any examples of counselling on wards, in your training, on video (simulations)?'

With the exception of informal consent, I've only ever seen counselling being botched.

As mentioned previously access to counselling has been minimal over the five years. Occasionally I have seen senior doctors [in relevant fields] offer advice [e.g. in hospices with the terminally ill]. In respect to videos, these are shown in the lectures, and if these are not attended [as they are often not compulsory] a student may not witness an expert in action.

I've seen examples of counselling, not on wards but in training videos.

There were training situations available for each of these situations e.g. seminars, small group teaching, videos. These come at the end of the second year.

I have observed numerous examples of counselling in my general training on the wards and in clinics, but on video on only a few occasions.

It appears that these students have to rely on observation and modelling to develop their counselling skills rather than through specific and structured teaching and learning experiences. Observation and modelling can be very effective techniques for learning counselling skills if the role models have sufficient expertise and can demonstrate good practice. These techniques are equally effective for inculcating bad practice.

LINKING PRIMARY AND SECONDARY
MENTAL HEALTH CARE

Drawing on their experiences at the Liverpool Psychotherapy and Consultation Service, Bill Barnes (Clinical Director) and Dr Michael Göpfert (Consultant Psychotherapist) envisage a coherent system of primary and secondary mental health care for the future (Göpfert and Barnes 1994). Recognizing that a 'counsellor-shaped gap' has been identified in primary care, Göpfert and Barnes stress the importance of training and professional role development for counsellors; training for GPs and other professionals working in primary care in psychological aspects of their work; and use of their own specialist psychotherapy and consultation service as an umbrella organization to manage the provision. This service would facilitate a network of support for counsellors providing supervision and auditing the counsellors' professional development.

Initial responses to a consultation document outlining this strategy were positive but showed that the dominant frame of reference was the *referral culture*, concerned with who refers to whom. Göpfert and Barnes summarize this issue as an assumption:

> that a problem is located in the patient rather than allowing space for the possibility that it may partly reside between patient and doctor. Were medical training to help students to clarify further their relationship to the 'psychological', doctors might use counsellors and psychotherapists differently . . . The professional role development part of our training strategy would run counter to the referral culture in that our counsellors would become carriers of an alternative 'consultation culture' within primary care in psychologically minded and non-psychologically minded practices alike.
>
> (Göpfert and Barnes 1994:12)

The authors envisage Acute Psychiatry provision being more clearly defined as a crisis service. The Psychotherapy and Consultation Service, in addition to coordinating primary care counselling and maintaining a collaborative dialogue with community mental health teams, would also be responsible for providing a secondary care non-crisis therapy service for people having serious but containable difficulties.

HOSPICE CARE

The philosophy of hospice care is very old. Its early associations were Christian, for example, the Knights Hospitallers of the Order of St John, who organized hospice care for wounded and dying Crusaders. This work was continued in monastic settings. When we lived more closely with death, care of the dying was a very significant part of everyday life. This emphasis has shifted with our increasing capacity to cure disease and prolong life. As provision of hospital care grew in line with growth in medical treatments, special provision for the dying declined.

Its renaissance is due to pioneers, like Dame Cecily Saunders who founded St Christopher's Hospice in Kent in 1967, in an attempt to counteract the imbalance between the progress being made in medical ability to save lives and the standstill in controlling the pain and distress of patients who were dying. The hospice movement in the UK now consists of about 50 hospices with highly trained and experienced staff devoted to maintaining the dignity and comfort of their patients. Hospices tend to be small, between 12–25 beds for in-patient care and some additional facilities for day care. Their central aim is to care for patients at the end of their lives, but this work was extended as hospices began to offer counselling for the families of their patients. Volunteers were recruited to offer bereavement counselling as an outreach provision, visiting relatives in their own homes.

Hospice care is holistic care, holistic in terms of the patients' needs – both physical and emotional – and holistic in its combination of medical treatments – research and teaching – especially in the areas of pain and symptom control and counselling. There is usually a higher nurse/patient ratio than in general hospitals and fewer doctors. The movement has attracted a great deal of public support and lay and voluntary staff are involved in helping to run hospices, in providing additional counselling support and raising funds. The need to combine expert palliative medicine with the need of patients and their families to talk about what is happening is well expressed in the hospice movement.

WHERE DOES COUNSELLING FIT INTO MEDICAL SETTINGS?

We have already seen that counselling is a complex and often bewildering process. Breakwell's (1987) mapping exercise for BAC showed that there was a wide range of definitions of counselling in medical settings and considerable confusion about what it meant. Since counselling is still used to cover a range of activities, from selling cosmetics to a stage in the disciplinary procedure for nurses, perhaps this is not so surprising.

Questions such as, 'What is counselling?' and 'What are the differences between counselling and psychotherapy?' have a heightened significance in medical settings (see Figure 2.1 showing the overlapping nature of counselling and psychotherapy). Such questions are linked to the three threads of lay, traditional and scientific medical treatments and to the dilemma of where counselling fits into the dominant paradigm of the medical model. It is also linked to the past and to the roots of counselling and psychotherapy. Although Freud was medically trained and construed himself as scientific, his education, typical of his time, also included philosophy and literature. It was not Freud's intention that psychoanalysis be welded to medical practice, even if he did hope for his theories to be one day capable of a physiological description (Jacobs 1984).

The confusion about where counselling fits arises from the narrowing of medical training as much as from the process of counselling itself. Sturgeon (1985) considers that one effect of the structure of medical education is that many students approach their clinical training thinking of patients as biological, biochemical systems with little control over the external or internal physical factors causing their illnesses. If students are taught by doctors who are primarily interested in scientific aspects of medicine, as Sturgeon points out, it is not surprising that they become dismissive of the psychological and psychosocial aspects which are under-played or ignored. Students have brief introductions to psychiatry with emphasis on diagnosis, treatment and management of classically presented psychiatric illnesses (Wolff *et al.* 1985).

Much in line with this warning about reductionism, Charlton (1993) argues for a return to a more holistic education for medical students as a preparation for working with patients in the context of their whole lives rather than a training which concentrates only on medicine and medical morality, skills and knowledge. Seale and Pattison (1994) think that current trends in medical curricula and textbooks do show a move towards new models of professional behaviour which incorporate understanding of psychological and sociological influences. They claim that medical students are now learning to be much more conscious of the way they communicate with patients. What do our group of young medical students have to say about this? Responding to the question, 'In what ways has your training prepared you for counselling patients and their families,

Nature of provision	Befriending/ Supporting	Using counselling skills of listening and responding with genuineness, empathy and respect	Counselling is concerned with helping clients to focus on and deal with current problems in their lives	Psychotherapy is concerned with the resolution of long-standing personal issues	Psycho-analysis focuses on gaining understanding and insight about how relationships in the past are being re-enacted in the present
Typical time-span	Can range from one contact to life-long support (usually short term)	Brief	Short term	Long but can be brief and focal	Long
Contact time	Varies – irregular	Varies – irregular, spontaneous, embedded in other activities	Typically weekly for up to an hour at an agreed time	1 or more sessions of 50 mins a week at agreed, contracted times	3–5 sessions of 50 mins a week at agreed, contracted times
Providers	Volunteers and paid/ unpaid co-ordinators of drop-in centres, self-help groups, patients groups, telephone/letter lines	Potentially all staff employed or involved in medical settings	Counsellors, Counselling psychologists	Psychotherapists	Psychoanalysts, Analytical Psychologists
Qualifications	Time, energy, commitment, under-standing, capacity for concern	For primary occupational identity. May also have counselling qualifications	In Counselling/ Psychology to BAC/ BPS or equivalent levels of accreditation	In Psychotherapy to UKCP or equivalent requirements for registration	Institute of Psychoanalysts. Society of Analytical Psychologists

Figure 2.1 The overlapping nature of counselling and psychotherapy

for example with death and dying, post-traumatic stress, depressions, suicidal tendencies?' They replied:

> Counselling as such hasn't been formally taught but time has been spent on communication skills in general. Everyday exposure to death and dying probably gives you greater life skills than someone of the same age would otherwise have. Training gives you the ability to provide information (e.g. prognosis, management) about the latter three but there's no specific help for counselling.

> The medical school tries to involve the students in group sessions for counselling such groups. But in what is an already overcrowded syllabus, it appears only lip service has been paid to this topic in the five years, and I would definitely NOT feel confident counselling any of the groups mentioned. With depression often seen on psychiatric attachments, there has been some contact with such patients. But this is often in the context of diagnosis and treatment (mainly pharmacological), not counselling.

> Few seminars, no formalized training. Hard to know how well one will cope when faced with situations.

> I haven't come into contact with breaking bad news about death, depressions and suicidal tendencies – in psychiatry it was useful as you knew what to expect.

> My formal medical training (i.e. actual specialist lectures or seminars) has prepared me rather poorly for counselling. Counselling patients and families on death and dying has been covered formally on a few occasions, but post-traumatic stress, depression and suicidal tendencies have only been discussed as formal medical topics as part of my psychiatry attachments. Although I have studied the aforementioned topics and have seen appropriate patients, I have not had training in how to offer counsel to them.

We know too much about psychological influences to ignore them. If medical staff feel that counselling competence is outside the limits of their own experience they should be able to refer to colleagues for alternative provision. The feelings expressed by a parent after her disabled daughter's death (Kahtan and Fitton 1993) vividly describe and highlight this need.

> We wish that someone had taken time to talk all this through with us before she died just so that we knew what to expect

and why it was happening that way . . . medical students should be taught about communication. They should have to see people with common problems in their exams and they shouldn't become doctors unless they have shown an ability to cope . . .

What is needed is a shared language. Greater understanding of counselling as a distinct process with underlying theoretical principles and codes of practice, can influence the way that questions about its effectiveness are framed and investigated and ultimately also influence questions about its place in medical settings.

· THREE ·

The practice of counselling in medical settings

THE ROLE OF THE COUNSELLOR

As the BAC Guidelines for the Employment of Counsellors in General Practice make clear, defining the counsellor's role is crucial. This is so across the whole range of medical settings and is essential if counselling is to be monitored and evaluated. The key areas of the counselling role will need to be clarified: defining the client group; accepting and making appropriate referrals; maintaining departmental, unit or practice records; and liaising with other staff. This clarification is especially important where counselling is part of a wider occupational or job specification. The counsellor's role may also be educative, raising awareness and understanding of the counselling process and the use of counselling skills in others, and possibly providing training placements and supervision for trainee counsellors. Any or all of these aspects are likely to involve the counsellor in issues relating to ethical codes, confidentiality, boundaries, and potential role conflicts. The counsellor's training, experience and competence should be adequate for the various aspects of the role within medical settings.

TRAINING AND QUALIFICATIONS

As part of a national initiative to improve the number and level of qualifications among the workforce the government established a new organization, the National Council for Vocational Qualifications (NCVQ), to oversee the development of qualifications linked to occupational standards. Financial support was provided through the Employment Department for representatives from industry to determine standards of competence for their particular vocational area. These representatives formed groups called Industry Lead Bodies. The Advice, Guidance and Counselling Lead Body was established in 1992 to set standards and qualifications for all those (both specialist and non-specialist) employed in advice, guidance or counselling, irrespective of job or status. By 1994 psychotherapy had joined the Lead Body which was then entitled The Advice, Guidance, Counselling and Psychotherapy Lead Body. The new qualifications will all be expressed in terms of the competences required for working in advice, guidance, counselling and psychotherapy at various levels. The British Association for Counselling (BAC) and the British Psychological Society (BPS) already have their own accreditation processes, which are likely to be adapted eventually to match those qualifications approved by the NCVQ. The BAC Guidelines for the Employment of Counsellors in General Practice make a strong recommendation to general practitioners to employ only those counsellors who have completed relevant training and achieved such standards. If counsellors are employed while still working towards achieving these standards there should be an agreed time scale for completion, linked to a future contract of employment. The Counselling in Medical Settings Division of BAC also recommends that staff employed as counsellors should have undertaken a recognized training. Staff whose work involves the use of counselling skills should be allowed time, funding and encouragement to be trained in basic counselling techniques and practice.

In Chapter 2 you met Su, Gilbert and Connor who described how their theoretical approaches influence their work with clients. All counsellors in medical settings should have experienced a period of formal training which integrated a coherent conceptual framework about human development with a consistent, theoretical approach and was well balanced with appropriate skills practice. If the counsellor uses an integrative approach there should be an understanding of why and how specific approaches are selected to match the needs of a particular client/client group at any one time. This is well illustrated in the following description from Darwin, a counsellor who uses such an approach.

DARWIN

I'm actually employed as a nurse teacher, a specialist subject leader in behavioural sciences, communications and interpersonal skills.

Counselling is a small but important part of my main role. My
manager encourages me to maintain a caseload in order to keep up
my clinical competence; I see an average of three clients a week and
I also supervise trainee counsellors. My clients are people who have
been referred to the Community Mental Health Team by their GP
or they might arrive via Occupational Health. I see some staff too.
I have autonomous clinical responsibility if people self-refer but if
referral is through the Community Mental Health Centre the Consultant Psychiatrist has responsibility. After an assessment session I
always negotiate a contract with the client. I don't see everyone for
a set amount of sessions: sometimes it's six weeks, it can be as long
as three years.

Linking my theoretical ideas with my training makes me think
of it as a natural history of where I am now. How I got to where
I am. How I work today. I work integratively. My training on my
Diploma Course at York was very strongly biased towards Gerard
Egan's Skilled Helper, a problem management approach, and I think
it was useful to get a really good grounding in one approach, so that
I felt competent in that way of working before moving on to use
other ways. Since then I've completed my M.Ed. in Counselling. It's
not a requirement to be trained or qualified as a counsellor for my
job but it's important to me. I feel ambivalent about the usefulness
or relevance of my medical background. It is useful to have had a
long contact with the systems but it's minimally useful, inhibiting
even, in terms of the presenting issues.

I think initially the way I worked with Egan, and still do sometimes, is that it's very much a map that guides the journey and
something I can refer to when I feel lost. Gradually, as I've had
further experience and done more training, I've become familiar
with other theoretical models and the question I most often ask
myself now is, 'What's the most helpful thing to do with this client
at this time given their resources?' I suppose what I like to do is to
pick up my cues from the client. Almost instinctively now, I like to
listen to the language that they use and the way they describe
where they are. From that I pick up cues as to what kind of things
might be helpful for them. Let me give you an example.

I was working with someone last week – I haven't been working
with her for very long – and I noticed that the way she described
where she was in terms of different parts of herself, as if these
existed as different people. My instinct was to follow that – try to
work with that – I suppose it was a more Gestalt way of working
with her. I think the language clients use and the way I experience
them in the encounter leads me down certain routes with them.

What I think underpins all this and makes it safe is that I feel I have a grounded knowledge of different approaches.

The safety net is that the core conditions of the relationship are in place. Then I think it's safe practice to follow the client's leads. In terms of responsibility I see it as me having responsibility for the space and process and the client having a responsibility for the content. Clients bring what they bring and I follow whatever seems to be helpful at that moment. Certainly in short-term work that tends to be influenced by my work with Egan, but what I've found as I've become more confident in my work is that I don't necessarily have a theoretical approach or model right at the front of my mind. I'm not saying I don't work with theory, what I am saying is that it's less prominent, it's become part of my nature, part of the way I counsel. I think a model is only useful in so far as it helps to improve a person's quality of life, so it isn't more important than the client. Sometimes people try and make the client fit the theory rather than thinking about how the theory can serve the client.

Past, present, future, my preference is to take cues from the client – what would be the most helpful thing to help this client at this time, that is my fundamental rule. Supervision of course helps with that – if you're using a whole variety of ideas it's really important to have the space to discuss them. Currently I am swinging back more to psychoanalytic ideas and I think that stems from the supervision work I do. Ideas I've moved away from in the past tend to be much more at the front of my mind as I'm working now.

I try not to – I'm aware of the dangers of a cookbook approach to counselling – look in the recipe book and get something out. It is important to understand the world view, the psychology, the philosophy behind those techniques so that I'm not just using them 'off the shelf'. The way someone describes a situation leads me to work in a certain way. That brings to mind Kelly's work – if you understand the goggles people see the world through that's as important as understanding what they are going through – so if you know their phenomenal field – or the way they make sense of the world – that gives you a clue as to how they work. It is existentially impossible to stand in someone else's shoes but you can certainly get in tune with some of the ways that they make sense of the world. I'm listening very carefully to that as well as to the content. What kind of language, what kind of non-verbal communications is the client using, would it be helpful to not always use words but also some dramatic, more creative approaches?

Darwin's account shows the relevance of ongoing training and personal development for counsellors and his capacity to be a reflective practitioner. The development of national vocational qualifications (NVQs) by the Lead Body for Advice, Guidance, Counselling and Psychotherapy offers an opportunity to more clearly define and recognize the competence and expertise of counsellors at different stages of their professional development. This should help to clarify some of the confusion surrounding the plethora of different qualifications and approaches and help managers and employers in medical settings to get a clearer picture of what counsellors actually do, especially since NVQs offer access to written statements of the competences required for qualifications at different levels. It is a requirement of BAC that its members adhere to its *Code of Ethics and Practice for Counsellors*, including the need to 'take all reasonable steps to monitor and develop their own competence'.

ETHICAL ISSUES – CODES AND STANDARDS OF ETHICS

Counsellors in medical settings draw on a range of codes of practice to help them make ethical decisions. Codes of Standards and Ethics for counsellors are available for members of the British Association for Counselling, British Psychological Society and British Association for Sexual and Marital Therapy. In addition, the majority of health care staff also work within medical ethical guidelines produced for specific professional groups by organizations such as the General Medical Council, the United Kingdom Central Council for Nursing, Midwifery and Health Visiting and the British Medical Association.

We may desire and expect counsellors to be persons of integrity who wisely follow the dictates of their informed consciences and always act in the best interests of their clients. This is too vague and ambiguous to be a sufficient guide to good practice. Nor does access to medical ethical codes necessarily mean that dilemmas in counselling are made any easier to resolve. It does, however, mean that there is a framework in place to guide thinking about a particular situation that can be adapted to fit counselling in medical settings. Medical ethics in general involves a consideration of moral philosophy, the law, the resources available and what practitioners want in practice; this is also true of ethics in counselling (Bond 1993; Jenkins and Gillon 1993).

The general ethical principles of moral philosophy, (autonomy, beneficence, non-malificence and justice) have no legal status and none of them are absolutes so that each must be considered in the light of the others. As Bond points out, moral philosophers have not shown a significant interest in counselling to date, probably because of lack of clarity about the counselling role. Research into counselling in medical settings has followed the dominant scientific paradigm of its context rather than examine questions of moral values. This is an area of potential conflict, especially when medical expertise is used as a power base to decide on forms of treatment available, for example, between drugs or counselling. When people are prescribed essential long-term medication they may still benefit from counselling. 'Whatever form of treatment is offered should rely on listening to establish the person's individuality and the place where they are coming from. They should respect that in "confused states" people can have a sense of their own needs', stated one person diagnosed as mentally ill (Wood 1993:19). MIND recommends the availability of independent advocates to help people to make decisions about whether counselling is right for them, whether the approach is suitable and to help resolve ongoing issues. MIND argue that this could be funded from a proportion of fees paid for training and membership of professional bodies.

Patients' Charters are part of the consumerist trends being promoted in the National Health Service of the 1990s. Seale and Pattison (1994) report that there is evidence that authoritarian approaches which infantilize and reduce choice and autonomy are being counteracted by more recent training in models of behaviour which emphasize patient-centred interaction. However, their view that training in communication and counselling skills are increasingly being included in initial training was not altogether confirmed by the responses from the young medical students in Chapter 2. When asked about their understanding of the ethical issues involved in counselling, one student gave the cryptic comment, 'Complex!' The others responded a little more fully:

> In acting as a counsellor, I believe that the most important ethical issue involves ensuring that your personal opinions do not influence the information given. A patient seeking counsel must receive the appropriate information in an unbiased manner.

> How much should you tell them/should they know, versus how much do you *want* to tell them, versus how much do they *want* to know?

Ethical issues of counselling seem primarily concerned with confidentiality. In order to counsel a patient it is often necessary to obtain information of a delicate and sensitive nature e.g. drug taking, previous sexual offences, etc. This information has often being obtained through the development of mutual trust. But should this information be of any legal importance, to betray the trust of the patient may prove to be more damaging in the long term to all concerned.

Complex – areas of confidentiality in illegal matters.

Patient-centred training encourages autonomy and consequent adult-to-adult consultations, with patients in partnership rather than in compliant roles. Experts, including counsellors and psychotherapists, may know more about technical issues but that does not necessarily qualify them to make moral judgements, or to make such judgements by themselves. Counsellors in medical settings have a valuable educative function in showing an alternative way of working which respects peoples' own version of what is 'good for them'; does not make assumptions, and regards them intrinsically as having equal rights and status in the process. Similarly, the counsellors own self-respect for their autonomy must also be taken into account. Counsellors are not absolutely obliged to do what a client wants. Actions which go against the counsellor's own moral principles, the law or professional codes of conduct may be refused. Darwin describes his experiences of liaison with his clients' referrers and some of the dilemmas with which he is faced:

If the client is referred by the Community Mental Health Team I have to give feedback. This can be notes on attendance and general progress rather that the confidential content of the sessions. It's a more sensitive situation with staff. I keep my feedback to a minimum then. Managers sometimes try to ferret out information about staff. This has increased since the Clothier Report. Mental health problems are a real taboo subject.

The principle of beneficence, to achieve the greatest good, is about producing net benefit over harm rather than an attempt to avoid harm at all costs. The question of whether counselling always benefits clients is pertinent. Wood's (1993) report for MIND encodes this question in its title, *Wordswordswordswords, the Power of Words: Uses and Abuses of Talking Treatments*. The report acknowledges that counselling and psychotherapy can be effective in alleviating distress and recommends that they be made more widely available if steps can be taken to ensure safe practice and the providers made more accountable.

In its policy paper on primary care MIND (1993) recommends in-creased access to counselling via every general practice; improved access to psychotherapy services and reduced budgets for psychotropic drugs. These recommendations are supported by evidence from the MIND survey that dissatisfaction with psychotropic medication was high because of adverse side effects. Where counselling and psycho-therapy were available, they were more popular than other treat-ments. Seventy-five per cent of the sample in the survey who were in psychotherapeutic relationships reported that they were satisfied or very satisfied with their treatment. A Mori Poll commissioned by the Royal College of Psychiatrists indicated that 91 per cent of the general public believes counselling to be the best response to de-pression (MIND 1993).

Non-maleficence is usually considered in conjunction with bene-ficence and is concerned with a duty to do no harm. Counselling and psychotherapy do carry a potential risk of causing harm to clients and their families. One of psychotherapy's most adamant critics, Jeffrey Masson (1989) would claim that it is inevitably harmful and abusive. There is clearly a contradiction between Masson's views and the consumer feedback from the MIND and Mori surveys. Clients often feel worse before they feel better and their capacity to sustain themselves through the often painful process of counselling or psychotherapy must be given proper consideration at initial as-sessment. Repression is sometimes merciful and the breaking down of defences can be traumatic and disturbing. Getting in touch with feelings previously cut off can be frightening rather than exhilarat-ing and liberating. The stages of dependency and regression that clients might undergo can leave them alarmed and fragile. There can, for some people, be a risk of breakdown and suicide. There may be conflict between benefits to the clients (more freedom, independence, assertiveness) and a possible negative effect of this on existing relationships. This principle has to be linked to the therapeutic arena. The issue of beneficence for the individual client is paramount in individual therapy, the couple in couple work while in family therapy, the family group is the primary concern.

The principle of justice, the fair distribution of resources and respect for the rights of others and the law raises some interesting points when applied to access to counselling and psychotherapy within the National Health Service. As Wood's (1993) study points out, there were an estimated 100,000 Britons receiving psycho-therapy in 1993, many of these in NHS settings, but with no evi-dence that provision was allocated on the basis of greatest need. People diagnosed as having mental illness were found to be most usually offered treatment with drugs; there was an 11,000 long waiting list for appointments with a clinical psychologist. In 1993 only about 33 per cent of all general practitioners had counsellors attached. This same study showed that the availability of psycho-therapists and counsellors had increased for clients living in the South-East of England which matched the findings of BAC's 1993 membership survey that there was a greater concentration of counsellors in this area.

NHS provision of talking treatments is very limited nationally and certain groups have far less access to therapy than others. According to MIND the most disadvantaged are black and minority ethnic groups, working-class people, lesbians and gay men and the elderly. These same groups are further disadvantaged because they are less likely to be able to pay for therapy outside the NHS thus restricting their access to independent counsellors and psychotherapists (Wood 1993).

One area of counselling in medical settings in which ethical issues are involved with statutory requirements is the field of assisted conception. The Human Fertilization and Embryology Act (1990) was introduced in response to moral and ethical concern regarding the use of gamete donation and *in vitro* fertilization, and legislated for the establishment of a statutory-based counselling service with its own Code of Practice. This Code requires BAC accreditation as a statutory minimum requirement for counsellors working in regulated clinics if they are not chartered psychologists or qualified social workers. If the staff are not qualified to this level the code requires access to such a person for staff and clients. The BAC's (1993a) *Code of Ethics and Practice for Counsellors* offers general guidelines regarding legal requirements advising that:

- (B.2.6.1) Counsellors should work within the law and;
- (B.2.6.2) Counsellors should take all reasonable steps to be aware of current legislation affecting the work of the Counsellor. A counsellor's ignorance of the law is no defence against legal liability or penalty.

Counsellors in medical settings have to work in the borderland of professional codes and guidelines and personal morality. Sometimes dilemmas can be resolved by adherence to statutory requirements, but there are times when the counsellor must handle the tension of having a foot on either side of the border. There is a moral/ethical dimension in much of the developmental work on the frontiers of medical knowledge which was not so in the early days of medical research. Questions now revolve not just around 'can we do this?' but *should* we do this?' Developmentally, moral and ethical thinking is frequently out of step with technical expertise.

CONFIDENTIALITY

Confidentiality is a central issue in the organizational and personal ethical codes of all counsellors and counselling relationships. It is the padlock on the chain of all the other linked issues such as supervision, settings, boundaries, record and note keeping and access to information. Confidentiality makes links with other health care staff and agencies more secure and ensures, as far as possible, sufficient safety for the counselling relationship to be based on that most critical feature of counselling, trust. A counselling relationship without trust is a contradiction – it is not a counselling relationship. Trust is a core condition for risk-taking, disclosing, revealing and exploring personal intimate thoughts and feelings with another person. Unlike many other procedures in medical settings, counselling is not something we do to our clients that requires only their compliance, it is a way of being with them that requires their active participation in the process.

In addition to difficulties raised by the complex nature of implementing ethical practice, there are a number of additional links in the chain of health care settings that affect confidentiality. The brief outline of ethical issues above demonstrates that there are no absolutes but there are some guiding principles. By its very nature, counselling in medical settings implies that the counsellors work within a team of people for whom a flow of communication is essential in order to provide consistent medical care. This in turn implies that relevant information will be shared. Practical and ethical issues come together in the central question of how confidentiality can be maintained while at the same time team members are able to communicate and co-operate with each other, as the following examples demonstrate.

CASE STUDY

Verity works as a counsellor in a primary health care centre set on the outskirts of a large industrial town. There are a total of 19 staff in the team: six general practitioners; a practice manager; two practice nurses; three receptionists/administrative staff; two health visitors; a medical secretary; a community outreach social worker; two community psychiatric nurses (employed by the District Health Authority) and Verity. Because of the high level of trust that already exists between staff and patients at the health centre, Verity finds that her clients understand and consent to her being able to discuss their progress with the doctors who retain overall clinical responsibility. This allows Verity and her clients to maintain confidentiality within a boundary which is made explicit at the outset of their contract. In the leaflet which outlines the nature of the counselling service and in her initial contact with clients, Verity considers how she can help them to understand the maintenance of confidentiality within this setting.

When she first started to work at the centre, Verity's colleagues found her different way of working very odd; she had to explain the meaning and significance of working in 50-minute sessions at regular times with no calls or interruptions during a session, in a room that was not also a storage space for leaflets and health promotion posters. Reception and nursing staff found it hard at first to understand how Verity could finish a session with some of her clients when it was obvious that they were in distress and that she gave very different responses when they asked if her clients were getting better. Because Verity sometimes made referrals to psychotherapy and psychiatric services, some staff thought that she was not fully competent, especially since she had a supervisor.

As part of her educative work with the team Verity has talked a great deal with her colleagues to enable them to understand the confidential nature of the content of her work with clients, what she means by boundaries, and why these are essential to counselling. Verity has found a way of allowing her clients to be in a private confidential space without her position in the primary care team being compromised. This enables her to take part in team discussions and case conferences and maintain her code of confidentiality.

On her part, Verity is careful to liaise with the reception and administrative staff, co-ordinating her diary with them. She has also worked with them to devise an efficient system for booking regular times, dealing with cancellations and getting in touch with her clients if necessary. Team meetings are not the only channel of communication between Verity and her colleagues. She contributes, as do all of the others, in the informal but important exchanges that occur over tea-making or in the reception area. Verity is secure enough in her role to take part in the *ad hoc* contacts that characterize general practice and primary health care; she does not need to remain aloof to maintain confidentiality.

Verity's role is aptly summarized by what Marilyn Pietroni describes as working in the *rhythm* of general practice at the Marylebone Health Centre in North London and by Annalee Curran and Roger Higgs use of *jazz* as the metaphor to reflect the teamwork at their surgery in Walworth Road in South London. This reflects a sensitive interaction, co-ordination and integration around a common theme and purpose (see p. 129).

CASE STUDY

The Marylebone Health Centre, based in the beautiful crypt of an old church, is offered as a model of good practice in the NHS by MIND (1993) in its policy paper on primary care. This innovative service offers an opportunity for its clients to choose from a range of traditional and complementary medicines including osteopathy, acupuncture and massage therapy alongside stress classes, befriending, counselling and referrals to long-term psychotherapy (Pietroni 1993). Practical advice and help is also available for welfare problems such as housing. Because the centre has a community outreach worker able to provide continuous support to refugees and minority ethnic clients, a major cause of stress is reduced, that of repeatedly explaining their situation regarding benefits and housing to new and different people. The community outreach worker post is funded through the ancillary staff health promotion budget.

The Centre makes less use of drug therapies than other practices locally and nationally, and the budget for psychotropic drugs has been dramatically reduced to one-third of the £80,000 typically spent by an average general practitioner in a year. These savings are used to fund the alternative services. The Director of the Centre, Patrick Pietroni believes that many people who visit the inner city health centre need neither therapy nor drugs but a combination of befriending, listening and practical support (Wood 1993). The Centre operates a telephone helpline staffed by volunteers from the Patient Participation Group, who are vetted, trained and supervised by the staff of the Community Outreach Unit, and who sign a confidentiality statement.

Marilyn Pietroni works as a part-time counsellor and psychotherapist in the practice. She stresses the complexity of working in general practice with presenting issues that range from risk of suicide to embarrassment and fear of blushing in public and the flexibility that this range requires, necessitating the ability to move in time to the changing rhythms of general practice. This incorporates working with individual clients in one of three patterns: extended assessment (up to four sessions); brief work (one to approximately 12 sessions); or what she calls the 'psychiatric out-patients' model (once a month or every six weeks over 1–2 years. Liaison must take place around this work with the primary health care team and services have to be provided within a tight resource framework.

Working with individual clients, Marilyn Pietroni's priority is to help them to think carefully about their presenting issues. She concentrates on the person's expression of pain and pressure, on their special circumstances and how they see their own problems and situation. The feelings that the clients generate in her and the impact of their body language are, for Marilyn, important guides to understanding and precede any theoretical explanation, although she works mainly in a psychodynamic framework. She also accepts that part of her role is to help the primary health care team to think about what clients are presenting and how they can work co-operatively. Boundaries are important for Marilyn, for example, around time and having a regular room, but they have to be pliable enough to adapt to the context. The confidentiality boundary at the Marylebone Health Centre includes all of the clinical team but not the wider community team.

The *Code of Ethics and Practice for Counsellors* from BAC (1993a) includes statements which clearly assume the importance of confidentiality and the need to ensure that clients are informed of what the boundary of confidentiality will be for them and that their consent is given. Since 1991, as part of the Patient's Charter, every citizen has had the legal right to have access to their health records and to know that those staff working for the NHS are under a legal duty to keep the contents confidential. Counsellors working within the NHS have to consider the implications of their statutory requirement for their own note-taking, record keeping and personal boundary of confidentiality.

BAC's *Code of Ethics and Practice for Counsellors* (1993a) includes the following clauses on confidentiality:

B.4. Confidentiality: clients, colleagues and others

- B.4.1. Confidentiality is a means of providing the client with safety and privacy. For this reason any limitation on the degree of confidentiality offered is likely to diminish the usefulness of counselling.

- B.4.2. Counsellors treat with confidence personal information about clients, whether obtained directly or indirectly or by inference. Such information includes name, address, biographical details, and other descriptions of the client's life and circumstances which might result in identification of the client.

- B.4.3. Counsellors should work within the current agreement with their client about confidentiality.

- B.4.4. Exceptional circumstances may arise which give the counsellor good grounds for believing that the client will cause serious physical harm to others or themselves, or have harm caused to him/her. In such circumstances the client's consent to a change in the agreement about confidentiality should be sought whenever possible unless there are also good grounds for believing the client is no longer able to take responsibility for his/her own actions. Whenever possible, the decision to break confidentiality agreed between a counsellor and client should be made only after consultation with a counselling supervisor or an experienced counsellor.

- B.4.5. Any breaking of confidentiality should be minimized both by restricting the information conveyed to that which is pertinent to the immediate situation and to those persons who can provide the help required by the client. The ethical considerations involve balancing between acting in the best interests of the client and in ways which enable clients to resume taking responsibility for their actions, a very high priority for counsellors, and the counsellor's responsibilities to the wider community.

- B.4.6. Counsellors should take all reasonable steps to communicate clearly the extent of the confidentiality they are offering to clients. This should normally be made clear in the pre-counselling information or initial contracting.

- B.4.7. If counsellors include consultations with colleagues and others within the confidential relationship, this should be stated to the client at the beginning of counselling.

- B.4.8. Care must be taken to ensure that personally identifiable information is not transmitted through overlapping networks of confidential relationships. For this reason, it is good practice to avoid identifying specific clients during counselling supervision/consultative support and other consultations, unless there are sound reasons for doing so.

- B.4.9. Any agreement between the counsellor and client about confidentiality may be reviewed and changed by joint negotiations.

- B.4.10. Agreements about confidentiality continue after the client's death unless there are overriding legal or ethical considerations.

- B.4.11. Counsellors hold different views about whether or not a client expressing serious suicidal intentions forms sufficient grounds for breaking confidentiality. Counsellors should consider their own views and practice and communicate them to clients and significant others where appropriate.

- B.4.12. Special care is required when writing about specific counselling situations for case studies, reports or publication. It is important that the author either has the client's informed consent, or effectively disguises the client's identity.

- B.4.13. Any discussion between the counsellors and others should be purposeful and not trivializing.

Some useful guidelines on confidentiality already exist for counsellors in medical settings. Bond (1993) suggests that the Code of Practice which accompanies the Human Fertilization and Embryology Act (1990) could be used more widely as an example of good practice. The Code states: '6.24. A record should be kept of all counselling offered and whether or not the offer is accepted. 6.25. All information obtained in the course should be kept confidential . . .' This enables counsellors to maintain a record of counselling which is available to the clinical team while maintaining confidentiality about the content. The Code gives further guidance for cases of concern:

- 3.27. If a member of a team has cause for concern as a result of information given to him or her in confidence, he or she should obtain the consent of the person concerned before discussing it with the rest of the team. If a member of the team receives information of such gravity that confidentiality *cannot* be maintained, he or she should use his or her own discretion, based on good professional practice, in deciding in what circumstances it should be discussed with the rest of the team.

This is similar to the United Kingdom Central Council (UKCC) Code of Professional Conduct which requires nurses to 'Respect confidential information obtained in the course of professional practice and refrain from such information without the consent of the patient/client or a person entitled to act on his/her behalf except where disclosure is required by law or by the order of a court or is necessary in the public interest.' The real dilemma is in the defining of 'information of such gravity that confidentiality cannot be maintained', or deciding when disclosure is 'necessary in the public interest'.

The Tarasoff case is often quoted as an example of just such a dilemma. A psychotherapist in America was told by a client that he was going to kill his ex-girl friend. The psychotherapist disclosed this to his superior and recommended that his client be compulsorily admitted to hospital. This did not happen for a variety of reasons and the client did murder his ex-girl friend. The victim's parents sued for damages and in the court case which followed two of the three judges ruled in favour of the view that the client should have been hospitalized and the girl friend and her parents warned of the threat. Codes of ethics and professional guidelines cannot make moral decisions for us, however much we may long for them to offer such precision. What they can do is to require us to commit ourselves to due and serious consideration of the principles embodied within them. Counsellors in medical settings will not find the 'right' answers to dilemmas concerning confidentiality in codes and guidelines but will find guidance to assist them in determining their own practice.

SUPERVISION

When counsellors and counselling psychologists recognize and adopt a professional code of practice and ethics, such as BAC's, it is considered unethical to practice without regular and ongoing supervision throughout their careers. The notion of supervision can be misleading and confusing to other staff in medical settings, especially if they equate it with apprenticeship or unqualified status. Supervision is about monitoring, developing and supporting counsellors so that the needs of the client are continually addressed. The BAC *Code of Ethics and Practice for the Supervision of Counsellors* (1988) covers the nature of the supervision process, the issues of responsibility and competence of the supervisor and the code of practice.

Employers in medical settings need to be aware of the nature and function of supervision and ensure that suitable arrangements have been made. It is particularly important that employers recognize that supervision is an essential aspect of the counsellor's job and that time and funds are allocated for this purpose. Supervision is about maintaining standards. It does have a monitoring and evaluation function but it serves a much broader purpose. In order to work effectively and creatively with clients, the counsellor needs to be able to explore alternative ideas in a supportive framework. This support is vital. In the regular space and time of supervision the counsellor is able to use the structure, as well as the content, in much the same way that the client uses the counselling relationship. In fact, the parallel process of client–counsellor and counsellor–supervisor are integral to reaching a better understanding of the counselling relationship. The BAC recommends a *minimum* of one-and-a-half hours of individual supervision per month, or the equivalent in group supervision, depending on the size of the group. Counsellors need to ensure that their supervision is adequate in proportion to the number of clients being seen each week.

Employers in medical settings usually maintain clinical responsibility for patients whom counsellors see on a regular basis as clients so it is important that employers, in addition to raising awareness and understanding among all medical staff about the role of counselling, also understand the role of the supervisor and preferably work in conjunction with supervisor and counsellor to ensure a quality service for clients. This could involve the employer, supervisor and counsellor in meeting to discuss their understanding of the supervision arrangements and to negotiate agreement on issues such as confidentiality. Furthermore, doctors could benefit from adopting a similar support system. In an article on 'Avoiding burnout in general practice', Chambers (1993) lists the factors contributing to stress and burnout, many of which could be alleviated if the stigma attached to needing help and support could be removed. The question 'Who cares for the carers?' is often asked and rarely answered satisfactorily. Regular supervision, in addition to its role in maintaining standards, is a way of building in professional support. The cost of this may be set against absenteeism, the personal costs of stress-related illness in carers and the pain and frustration caused to patients and clients when staff avoid the personally painful consequences of dealing with distress because no one deals with theirs. This point, which is emphasized in BAC's *Information Sheet* on supervision, could be equally applied to the whole range of medical services and practice:

> By its very nature, counselling makes considerable demands upon the counsellor, supervision helps to overcome some of the difficulties this creates. A counsellor can become over-involved or ignore some important point, or may be confused as to what is happening with a particular client. He may have undermining doubts about his own usefulness.
>
> (BAC 1990)

STAFF SUPPORT MECHANISMS

Consultative support (Bond 1993), in which counsellors use peers or an independent group leader to facilitate discussion about their practice, might be used in medical settings as an alternative to supervision. This has the advantage of shifting the focus of the relationship away from accountability, though it might generate its own confusion over the use of the word *consultancy*.

Informal and formal arrangements for peer consultancy and support are more common in medical settings. Formal schemes of GP and nurse training often involve the use of mentors, experienced staff who facilitate the trainee's progress towards qualified status (East 1995). The National Association for Staff Support (NASS) in its Charter for the Health Care Services (1992) advocates a proactive staff support policy. Recognizing the specific pressures generated by the stressful nature of working in health care and the high cost in terms of staff turnover, sickness and work performance with consequent effects on the quality of patient care, NASS urges recognition of staff support as an integral, legitimate and acceptable provision. NASS views the following principles as an essential part of any national or local staff support policy:

- Staff in health care services have individual rights to be valued and respected just as any other citizens have.
- Staff who are cared for provide the best quality of service; where there is inadequate care and support, staff will show high sickness, absenteeism and wastage rates.
- Staff are a valued and expensive resource. It makes good sense to maintain their fitness and capacity to give a good service in the interests of their personal job satisfaction and of maintaining the quality of patient care.
- A range of integrated services together with a general ethos of care is an essential provision. Also recognition of the nature of stress and of the need for emotional support in the workplace at all times is important.
- Identifying who is responsible for providing a stated policy, both nationally and locally, is necessary for co-ordination in all workplaces.

Such policy statements communicate the message that staff in medical settings need support, but many carers find it difficult to place their needs alongside those of their clients. Sometimes counselling provision is needed for medical personnel.

The National Counselling Service for Sick Doctors was established in 1985 to offer a confidential counselling service for doctors. Statistics show that doctors have higher rates of suicide, alcoholism, drug addiction and depressive illnesses than the average for the whole population. Women doctors are particularly liable to commit suicide (Rawnsley 1991). A complex array of factors are involved, including the stressful nature of being a doctor and so called 'medical personalities', characterized as high achievers and workaholics who tend to be obsessional and want certainty. A doctor's knowledge of drugs and ease of access to them can encourage dependency. Sick doctors in Rawnsley's study tended not to be registered with a general practitioner, had incomplete medical records, were defensive about admitting problems, reluctant to seek help and co-operate in treatments and had disdainful and dismissive attitudes about psychiatric and psychological problems. They did not seek help until they were desperate and very ill indeed. Doctors' wives in this study were frustrated that their husbands could not, or would not, share their feelings, that they worked extremely long hours and avoided conflict. The doctors had a tendency to prescribe medicine for their wives rather than talk to them. The suicide rate among doctors' wives is substantially higher than among doctors themselves and has risen during the past 20 years. This raises some interesting questions about doctors' preparedness to include counselling and psychotherapy within their range of provision for patients if it is outside their range of provision for themselves. It also demonstrates the stigma attached to having personal and emotional problems within the medical profession.

STIGMA

It seems that any word that starts with the prefix *psych* is liable to trigger off the kind of fear and anxiety that Hitchcock harnessed so well in the one word title of his film *Psycho*. The word *mental*, far from being a neutral descriptor for 'of the mind' is used in a variety of derogatory and threatening senses. This was clearly the initial response of a young client, Kay, when she received an appointment letter from her counsellor and saw that the address at the top of the headed notepaper said Mental Health Unit. In her initial interview Kay disclosed that she was very upset and frightened that people would call her *mental*.

In a blistering attack on 'our so-called caring systems', Brandon (1992) sets an ethical agenda to tackle the injustices and discrimination against people who have become overshadowed by their labels, particularly in the traditionally highly stigmatized areas of mental illness and mental handicap. When *care* has become *control*, counselling can be seen as a subversive activity which threatens the power of the carers by shifting the balance towards a consideration of the client's views. In an article that focuses on the therapist's counter transference in work with mentally handicapped clients, Symington (1992) raises the issue of 'unconscious contempt' in the therapist, noting the ways that clients suffer discrimination as a result. This may well have much wider significance, given the evidence about doctors' apparent contempt for their own psychological needs, in terms of decisions about resources for counselling services. A more open prejudice is displayed when insurance companies discriminate against customers who have been treated for depression and anxiety, with long-term implications for pensions. This has an unfortunate negative effect which may affect early diagnosis and prevent proper provision being made or inhibit take-up of the offering of counselling and psychotherapy if potential clients feel that this will lead to discrimination, prejudice and financial penalties.

If there is an underlying denial of need for counselling for the staff in medical settings how does this affect the provision for clients? The stigma that is attached to being seen to be in need of support, and to mental illness and mental handicap will be covered in more detail in the next chapter as we turn to some of the more specific issues in counselling in medical settings.

· FOUR ·

Specific issues in counselling in medical settings

Counselling in medical settings deals with as many issues as people are capable of experiencing in the endlessly complex and fascinating interplay of psyche and soma. Although counsellors using different theoretical models to underpin their work will place greater or lesser emphasis on these two aspects and the dynamic interaction between them, their counselling will involve working with people and their families or partners who are having difficulties in handling or coming to terms with illness, its treatment and its effects. This work may focus on feelings about specific physical conditions, mental health problems, reactions to bereavement and loss, and death and dying. Counsellors in medical settings also work with clients who feel ill or who present with physical symptoms of a disease when no disease can be located or diagnosed – when their bodies and minds have become the stage for a portrayal or dramatization of their feelings.

In order for counselling to be recognized as a distinct and separate process appropriate to deal with such issues, there are certain requirements that need to be fulfilled. This is true of counselling in all settings but particularly so in medical settings, because of the growth in this area and the pressure to justify this and any further expansion.

RESEARCH INTO COUNSELLING IN MEDICAL SETTINGS

Research into counselling in medical settings is a particularly important issue. Counselling needs to justify its existence, show it is giving value for money and show that it can make a significant contribution to the healing process. It would, as Scott and Marinker (1993) point out, be comforting if all changes in general practice could be based on reliable evidence from empirical research. They argue that even though there is a paucity of hard evidence to support their view, counselling is valuable because it fits the humane intentions of medical care.

The importance of investing in research and development for primary care has recently been recognized in the establishment by the Department of Health of a £15-million National Primary Care and Research and Development Centre. Over the next ten years the University of Manchester, in collaboration with the Centre for Health Economics at the University of York and the Public Health Research Centre at the University of Salford, will be mounting a comprehensive programme of research and development in primary care through the new National Centre. The cost effectiveness of counselling in general practice is one of the areas which will be tackled in the new Centre's research and development programme. The Department of Health has also prioritized the evaluation of counselling in general practice as part of its Health Technology Assessment Programme, as has the National Health Service Executive in its planning for a research programme to evaluate the cost effectiveness of counselling in primary care.

Counselling in medical settings has attracted a great deal of interest from researchers who have been investigating provision in order to evaluate its effectiveness. Table 4.1 gives a summary of some of the surveys and studies which have been carried out between 1975 and 1992. There is now a substantial body of evidence to show that clients, counsellors and doctors value counselling provision and can see benefits for individuals, their families and for the NHS in terms of reduction in the number of consultations and drug budgets. The beneficial nature of counselling in medical settings is now less in question than issues of priority and appropriateness, although there are some stern critics and cautious sceptics (Martin 1988; King 1994). Corney (1993) lists the main reasons why evaluative studies of the effectiveness of counselling in general practice are still essential and these apply to the whole range of counselling in medical settings. Evaluative studies are needed to identify which clients might benefit the most from counselling, given that decisions have to be made about prioritizing resources.

The question about the most appropriate use of resources lies behind investigative work with parents coping with the birth of a child with mental handicap. There are undeniable needs for staff

Table 4.1

Study	Method and Sample	Duration	Number of clients (and) number of sessions with counsellor	Presenting issues	Outcomes
Marsh, G.N. and Barr, J. (1975) Marriage guidance counselling in a group practice	Attachment of a marriage guidance counsellor to a group practice	Unknown	21 clients (couples) seen for average of 11 sessions	Relationship/ Emotional distress	Reduction in visits to GP. GPs increased detection in emotional and mental distress
Ives, G. (1979) Psychological treatment in general practice	Attachment of clinical psychologist to group practices	26 months and one year follow up	233 clients seen for an average of 5 × 1.5hr sessions (range of 1–20 sessions)	Anxiety Interpersonal problems Psychosomatic disorders	No change in referrals to psychiatrist. Reduction in GP consultation (36%) and in number of prescriptions issued for psychotropic drugs (50%) changes were maintained after one year follow-up
Anderson, S.A. and Hasler, J.C. (1979) Counselling in general practice	Questionnaires to first 80 patients using counselling service and their GPs (4). Additional information from medical records	3 months	80 clients (59% response) seen for an average of 5 times	Stress linked to crisis and trauma. Longer-term personal and social issues	Subjective – an improvement as measured by the feelings of patients and doctors. Majority of patients said they had been helped by counselling and would

Study	Method	Duration	Sample	Problems	Outcomes
			(15 attended group sessions)		recommend it to relatives or friends. Objective – reduction in prescriptions of psychotropic drugs and medical consultations
Waydenfeld, D. and Waydenfeld, S.W. (1980) Counselling in general practice	4 questionnaires for each recruited patient on data at outset and end of counselling; information from medical records for 6 months after counselling; patient evaluation 6 months after counselling; structured interviews with GPs; and written comments from counsellors	2 years	9 counsellors 35 GPs 99 clients seen for an average of 15.4 sessions, (range 1–114)	Anxiety Marital/ Relationship problems Sexual problems Psychosomatic symptoms	Patient feedback was positive Reduction in consultations (31%) Reduction in prescriptions Increase in number of working class patients having access to a counsellor
Martin, E. and Mitchell, H. (1983) A counsellor in general practice: a one-year survey	Questionnaires sent to 60 patients, 15 counselled for abortion were excluded. Remaining 12 had moved away. 70% response	1 year	87 clients seen for an average of 2.3 sessions	Anxiety/stress Marital problems Abortion	High proportion of failed first appointments and subsequent appointments (29%). Reasons – longer than average waiting time. Directed to counselling by GPs. 90% of respondents found counselling to be helpful

Table 4.1 (cont.)

Study	Method and Sample	Duration	Number of clients (and) number of sessions with counsellor	Presenting issues	Outcomes
Ashurst, P.M. and Ward, D.F. (1983) An evaluation of counselling in general practice	Random selection and allocation to either a counsellor or for routine GP treatment of patients who had consulted GP for a neurotic disorder – not necessarily seeking counselling	1 year	726 clients	'Neurotic' disorders	Patients valued counselling help but no striking differences were measured against the control group after one year, though authors noted that some individuals had benefited considerably
Martin, E. and Martin, P.M.L. (1985) Changes in psychological diagnosis and prescription in a practice employing a counsellor	(a) Practice sample. Random selection of 300 patient files – monitored for psycho-social problems and prescription of psychotropic drugs in 1975, 1979, 1982. (b) Patients consulting counsellor, a survey of notes	(a) Review of 7 years patient case histories (b) Review of referrals for psychiatric problems and prescriptions	(a) 300 patients continuously registered for 7 years (b) 87 clients who had attended counselling one year before survey	(a) All (b) Psycho-social problems	(a) Numbers of patients with psychiatric diagnosis fell from 16.3% to 10.6%. Psychotropic drugs increased by 3.7%. Anti-depressants fell by 17%. Tranquillizers and sleeping tablets increased by 30% (b) Consultations with GP fell by 5.6% in the year after seeing the counsellor.

	for 12 months commencing after first appointment with counsellor	and 87 age/sex matched controls	N/A	Overall consultations fell by 24.2%. Psychotropic drug prescription rose by 56% but 88% of this was due to 4 of the 87 (37%) took no psychotropic drugs in the year before or after seeing the counsellor. 4% increase in prescriptions of psychotropic drugs to control group. In February 1985, 78% of patients had not consulted the GP about psychiatric problems or been prescribed psychotropic drugs. Authors conclude that no major changes were detected over the 7-year period
Balestrieri, M. Williams, P. and Wilkinson, G. (1988) Specialist mental health treatment in general practice: A meta-analysis	Meta-analysis of 11 British studies	N/A	N/A	N/A	Competence of the counsellor is the most significant factor, not approach or form, though counselling appeared to be most effective for social functioning and behaviour therapy. Reduced contact

Table 4.1 (cont.)

Study	Method and Sample	Duration	Number of clients (and) number of sessions with counsellor	Presenting issues	Outcomes
					with psychiatric services. Treatment by specialist mental health professional was found to be 10% more effective than GP alone
Petterson, G. (1992) User views on counselling services	Qualitative study using group discussion facilitated by an independent facilitator and colleague taking notes and taping for accuracy	2 hours group discussion	8 clients each seen for 6 sessions	Variety – including recent sudden traumatic event; reaction to receiving disturbing information in abrupt manner in hospitals; and long term depression and drug dependency	High level of patient perception of benefits of counselling including reduction in prescribed medication and increase in ability to cope with anxiety and stress

| Corney, R. and Stanton, R. (Unpublished) Counselling patients with marital problems | Subjects given an initial psychiatric, social and marital assessment. Data retrieved from medical notes for previous 6 months. Random allocation to group receiving counselling or waiting list control group who were offered counselling after follow-up assessment at 6 months. | 1 year | 47 subjects | Marital | Ongoing. After 6 months those referred for counselling had made much more improvement than control group on scores measuring depression, self-esteem and marital adjustment |

sensitivity, privacy, information, time to ask questions, referrals for support and to be treated as an equal adult. This does not take away the pain of this experience but does afford dignity and respect to the child and parents. However, it is not possible to predict which parents would benefit from longer-term counselling (Ditchfield 1992). All parents in these circumstances who wish to should have the opportunity to talk with someone, in order to identify those who might benefit from longer-term contact. The issue of who decides whether counselling is needed and/or wanted brings us up against the fundamental counselling principle of voluntarism and, once again, the need to clarify the differences between support from staff trained in the use of counselling skills and those trained to be counsellors. Such distinctions are necessary in order to assess appropriate provision and to ensure validity in follow-up studies of efficiency and effectiveness.

Decisions about priorities will always be with us. Even if we do not make a decision, we have made a decision not to make one! Existential and practical decisions are a fact of our lives from the day we discover that we can say 'no'. Having a 'yes' and a 'no' is the basis of personal identity, autonomy and responsibility. Some of us are blessed with parents, teachers and other authority figures who allow us to develop those qualities within ourselves. If we are less fortunate we learn that authority and responsibility lie outside and we must always seek permission and approval for our actions from those in authority. This can, of course, lead to a certain amount of resentment if not outright resistance or rebellion. It is often an issue that clients bring to counsellors, and as counsellors we need to be able to tolerate our own existential anxieties about personal issues of authority and autonomy to be able to justify the decisions we make about their access to counselling services. The aim to provide counselling services on the basis of greatest need assumes that this can be satisfactorily measured. Decisions do have to be made, resources are not infinite and there are competing claims, but as Rudolf Klein, from the Centre for the Analysis of Social Policy has pointed out:

> There is no technological fix, scientific method or method of philosophic inquiry for determining priorities. Of course, the three Es – economists, ethicists and epidemiologists – all have valuable insights to contribute to the debate about resource allocation and rationing, though none of them can resolve our dilemmas for us . . . much of medicine is about the management of uncertainty, where research may roll back the functions of

ignorance but is never likely to eliminate totally the need for clinical discretion and the use of judgement in interpreting the evidence about efficacy and outcomes.

(Klein 1993:307)

This brings us back to the ideas on codes of practice and ethical guidelines that we examined in Chapter 3. Research and evaluative studies can help to inform our decisions but in the end the search for principles or techniques will not make them for us. Priority setting is a theme throughout health care systems. There is a complex interaction of historical influences and new initiatives and policies at national level which define priorities and targets at local levels and which in turn affect local interpretation of needs.

If need was a precise and measurable concept then priorities would be easier to divine and manage. In the spirit of partnership advocated in the Patient's Charter will the clients' needs for counselling be considered equally and alongside the medical professions judgement of that need? As Klein points out, those who benefit most from the existing provision, as providers or consumers, are a strong, concentrated and well organized pressure group for maintaining the status quo. New services such as counselling, which depend on the reallocation of funds, are more diffuse and less organized. If discussions about priorities in medical settings are dominated by particular voices then evaluative studies can play an important part in defining and establishing a need for counselling because they add timbre to its voice. Counsellors must be able to engage in collective argument and open, ongoing debate to which evidence from research contributes. Then the conflicts between competing values and preferences can be explored in a rational manner:

It is a concept of rationality which goes back to Aristotle and which puts the emphasis on finding 'good reasons' to justify decisions. And it is an approach which, I would argue, leads us out of the dead end of searching some overarching formula for determining priorities by directing our attention to the *structure* of decision making.

(Klein 1993:310)

To assist in arguments about resource allocation for counselling in medical settings clarification is needed about the wide range of therapies that are available and there is a vital need to know more about the best match of provision to benefit clients. The confusion about the range of different talking treatments has been a theme throughout earlier chapters. What is needed is less competitive and rivalrous comparison of the different therapies and a much more comprehensive body of information about the therapies, and their effectiveness, appropriateness, acceptability and availability for clients.

There is also a need for evaluative studies to inform us about training needs, levels of skills, competence and expertise required by counsellors in medical settings. The development of standards by the Lead Body for Advice, Guidance, Counselling and Psychotherapy should add to the evidence. MIND's research on the talking treatments (Woods 1993) supports the active involvement of users in professional and training bodies' decision-making processes, especially in relation to training, ethics and complaints procedures. MIND recommends the establishment of a compulsory published register of counsellors and psychotherapists which lists the code of ethics to which they adhere and from which they can be struck off for gross professional misconduct and legal steps introduced to prevent their further practice.

New qualifications, including the introduction of NVQs; five new Diploma in Counselling in Primary Health Care courses for practising counsellors sponsored by the Counselling in Primary Care Trust; postgraduate courses in Counselling in Primary Health Care at City University; and a one-year Counselling in General Practice course offered by the British Association of Psychotherapists (BAP); all signal an increased professionalization and recognition of counselling in medical settings. All of these initiatives have the potential to strengthen and increase the body of knowledge and understanding, including research and evaluative studies in this area. In addition to the increased number of trained and qualified counsellors in medical settings graduating from these programmes, they should also act as a stimulus for more provision and for progression to more advanced levels of training and qualification.

LOSS

Doctors may be able to cure physical symptoms, and this in itself is likely to leave the patient feeling more positive about doctors, viewing them as powerful and effective. However sometimes the physical illness or its treatment leaves patients with an acute sense of loss. This can be actual loss of a limb, an organ or a facility and sometimes a vaguer though not less intense sense of loss of health, or of a premature understanding of eventual loss of life and being faced with one's own mortality.

In a sense, all counselling in medical settings is linked to loss: the disabling and mutilating losses of accidents or surgical treatments; the loss of faculties and strength; the loss of a healthy self-image; of a child; of the hope of ever becoming a parent; or of having a future to plan. There may be a secondary loss of employment and with it the source of income, relationships, status and self-esteem, and the patterns of a working life. In all losses we face, consciously or unconsciously, our assumptions about immortality and the final loss of life itself.

As Elizabeth Kübler-Ross (1989) concludes, to work with someone we know is dying requires a certain maturity which can come only from experience. If we are to work as counsellors and therapists in any context, there must be a willingness to examine our own attitudes and feelings about death and dying, since every ending must deal with feelings of loss. However, this is particularly relevant for counsellors in medical settings where we must deal not only with the symbolic and metaphoric links but the reality of death. In spite of its inevitability and universality this is not, as we will see on p. 89, an aspect of medicine that is handled very well. When Kübler-Ross began her Interdisciplinary Seminar on Death and Dying in 1965, she and her class of students from the Chicago Theological Seminary decided that the best way to study death and dying was to ask terminally ill patients in hospital to be their teachers. When she asked the physicians of different services and wards for permission to interview a terminally ill patient, Kübler-Ross found that there were no dying patients in the hospital. This is a powerful indicator of how hard it was, and still is, to accept the idea of active involvement in the preparation for death. 'We are always amazed how one session can relieve a patient of a tremendous burden and wonder why it is so difficult for staff and family to elicit their needs, since it often requires nothing more but an open question' (Kübler-Ross 1989:241). It also requires a willingness to do nothing, when there is nothing to be done, except to listen.

THE PATIENT IN THE HEALER AND THE HEALER IN THE PATIENT

There is a potential danger in medical settings of an omnipotent denial and splitting of roles into patient and healer, the sick and the well. Aveline (1992) discusses the notion of the archetype of patient and healer within us all. When the tension of the ambivalence generated by this duality is too great, the archetype may split into opposite poles, either of which can then be projected on to others.

If the healer locates the 'patient in him/herself' within the patient and denies its existence within his or her own self, there can be no admission of feelings of weakness, or personal terrors associated with disease, suffering and death. Healers need to be in touch with both polarities in order to mobilize the healer within the patient. This awareness and understanding that we may all be capable of creating our own illnesses and our own recovery, is not well integrated into traditional medical education with its clearly divided roles of those in need of support and those who offer it.

At best counselling offers clients an opportunity to relinquish their passive patient roles and engage in a relationship which in itself promotes change and healing. This does not have to include specific knowledge and understanding of disease, though that could be an advantage in some situations. More central is the deceptively simple recognition and acceptance of another person's distress and suffering and the willingness to engage with that person.

SPECIALIST OR GENERALIST?

If psychotherapy is an 'academic orphan' (Aveline 1992) within medical studies, where does this leave counselling in the family tree? In its struggle to gain entry and acquire legitimate status counselling often appears in disguise, or is adopted by those with acceptable primary occupational roles within medical settings, such as nurses, psychologists, occupational therapists, medical social workers and health visitors.

In the primary sector of education teachers usually describe their work in terms of their pupils: their ages, personalities, aptitudes and abilities, their families and their neighbourhood, a holistic, pupil-centred perspective. Secondary school teachers characteristically begin a description of their jobs with a reference to their subject specialism, a subject-centred perspective. In much the same way counsellors in primary care settings tend to be generalists, though they may have a medical or social work background. In secondary care, counsellors and/or staff using counselling skills, tend to define or specify their role as being linked to a primary occupational identity together with additional information about the particular disease, medical condition or areas of work in which they specialize, for example HIV/Aids, cancer, haematology, abortion, post-traumatic stress or bereavement. This may be because counselling posts are resourced through alternative avenues of funding linked to charities or patient support groups. It could also be influenced by a cultural ethos and value system which is geared to diagnosis and treatment of disease and has yet to fully recognize counselling as a healing process in its own right.

There are potential advantages and disadvantages in both positions of generalist or specialist counselling, though some counsellors would argue that there is no difference. Table 4.2 summarizes the positions. Aveline (1992) adds to the debate on whether psychotherapists should have a prior qualification in one of the core health professions, in which he includes nursing, occupational therapy, art and drama therapy along with medicine, psychology and social work. He concludes that although talent as a psychotherapist is not found exclusively in any one professional group, a background in one of the core areas ensures that trainees will be familiar with ethical procedures and the signs and symptoms of major psychiatric illness. Aveline sees qualifications from other backgrounds as relevant, providing that special training in recognizing psychiatric illness and the effects of prescribed drugs is also completed. It is a requirement of the BAC's *Code of Ethics and Practice for Counsellors* (1993a) that counsellors be aware both of the limitations of their own competence and of their ability to make appropriate referrals, so some similar training for counsellors is advisable.

SUPPORT FOR STAFF

Tyndall (1993) points out that people considered as natural counsellors because of their existing role in dealing with people in difficulties, for example, doctors and nurses, often have ingrained patterns of caring behaviour which is about *doing* on behalf of another, and about problem-solving and taking action. They therefore find it difficult to adopt the more passive stance of *being* involved in counselling. When nursing staff are employed as counsellors they can find themselves struggling with role conflicts arising within themselves and with their colleagues and not being sure about where they belong, as Allie and Heidi discovered when they took on counselling roles.

Allie's post as nurse/counsellor in an obstetrics and gynaecology department has split funding. Her nursing salary, paid by the NHS trust is complemented by additional funding for her counselling from a major charity. Allie says that she is in an 'eternal dilemma' about her split role. Heidi works as a full-time perinatal loss counsellor in a large inner-city hospital in the North of England. She trained and worked as a midwife for 12 years before taking her

Table 4.2   Advantages and disadvantages in specialist vs. generalist counselling

Specialist counselling	
Potential advantages	*Potential disadvantages*
Possibility of holistic care increased	Might concentrate on specific aspects of disease rather than whole person
Greater awareness and understanding of the course of a disease and the effects of treatment	May only be available during medical treatments giving rise to role conflict, ambiguity
Can detect symptoms in addition to recognition of feelings	Sidetracking into taking action in order to avoid painful feelings
Realistic expectations	Working within medical hierarchy role defined by institutional expectations with possible implications for confidentiality
Halo effect of medical credibility	Trying to be all things to all people
Working in a team of staff	Isolation and rejection by the team
Supportive and educative role	Unconscious and conscious rivalry
More widely understood and accepted if linked to well established role	No dedicated space for counselling

Generalist counselling	
Potential advantages	*Potential disadvantages*
More clearly defined role likely to lead to less ambiguity	Isolation, loneliness, marginal role
Can concentrate on client's expression of feeling about their disease, condition	May defer too readily to medical knowledge and expertise
Not sidetracked into activity to deal with symptoms, physical effects of illness	May not recognize effects of medical treatment or symptoms of serious disease
	May have no say in assessments or referrals for counselling

Table 4.2 (cont.)

Generalist counselling	
Potential advantages	*Potential disadvantages*
Can offer an alternative/ complementary provision	Anxiety about secrets between counsellor and client can lead to hostility and spoiling of counsellors' work. 'Does it work?' asked a senior nurse manager 'this namby-pamby counselling lark'
Offers an opportunity to talk about medical/nursing staff and treatments without taking part	
Educative and supportive role for other staff	Confidentiality boundary may include medical/nursing staff
	Dumping of too painful aspects of work by other staff
	Role of counsellor may not be understood

present position. Heidi loves her job which she finds fulfilling and rewarding but which also leaves her feeling isolated and devalued by other members of her unit. 'They don't handle death very well on my unit', says Heidi, whose very presence seems to remind the staff of their 'failures'. Heidi works in a non-ideal environment where her role is denied, only really acknowledged when she is not there to fulfil it and the other staff have no one to contain their distress. For example, the leaflet she has produced about the counselling service is not distributed to patients and their families by the nursing staff. Although workshops with their emphasis on practical activities are well attended, the support group which Heidi set up in response to a need expressed by the staff, was initially poorly attended and then not at all. Staff prefer to make incidental contact with Heidi, 'by the way' or to have postscript conversations in cloakroom doorways or the middle of a busy ward. Heidi feels that the activities of the workshop help to counter and mask painful feelings of failure and helplessness whereas joining a support group may suggest a difficulty in coping that is busily denied.

This unspoken, unacceptable implication that joining a support group means not coping, not being able to deal with the job and this being visible to colleagues and managers is very significant. Medical staff and their managers frequently appear to be more sympathetic to the suggestion that patients should have access to a counsellor than to the suggestion that their staff should, even when tacit or even overt support is given to this idea. There is a contradiction between expressed policy and hidden feelings. In spite of the widely expressed concern about stress and burn-out underlying the aims of organizations such as the National Association for Staff Support, there is a persistent hidden agenda that nurses and doctors should be taught to be 'hard'. What sort of support are the young medical students from the North-East offered?

> I feel that personal support is non-existent within the formal medical setting. If help is required it is usually sought by talking informally to friends or peers.

> None – but then when would counselling stop? Friends who have been in similar situations would be available informally.

> It is often seen as a sign of weakness, and an inability to cope with the stress and strains of a medical career to seek help. Therefore most people would be reluctant to seek help from strangers (although professionals in such fields) and would therefore probably seek amateur advice from known confidants i.e. friends and relatives.

> Very little support – it's almost assumed that we can deal with things on our own.

> None that I know of apart from friends.

These students' experiences support Menzies-Lyth's (1961, 1988) findings on the way that social systems in hospitals evolve to defend against intolerable anxieties inevitably caused by the stress of working in medical settings. Menzies-Lyth found evidence of depersonalization, categorization and denial of the significance of the individual, which inhibited the development of relationships between nurses and patients. There is a conflict between explicit support for staff and implicit denial of the need for it or fear of the consequences of being seen to need support. Explicit support is demonstrated in the publication of *Health at Work in the NHS* (HEA 1992), a long-term initiative set up to support the national strategy for health which must be included in annual corporate contracts and business plans. Subsequent reviews will monitor the implementation of a health promotion strategy including the development of counselling and group support for workplace stress, bereavement and organizational change. Anxieties and fears about the consequences of needing

support are expressed in the numbers of enquiries received by occupational health staff about whether, in the light of the Clothier
Report (1994) following the Beverley Allitt case, being seen to receive counselling support will affect future employment prospects.
The *Allitt Inquiry* itself suggests that excessive use of counselling is
a contra-indication for acceptance into nurse training.

This conflict and ambivalence about recognizing the need for
counselling and support within medical settings shows the powerfully lingering effects of the stigma of mental illness, the fear of
burn-out and the fear of being unable to cope among the professional super-copers. The need to improve mental health services
has been recognized as a key area in the Government's health
strategy. The attitudes of staff working within medical settings will
have a significant effect on the outcomes of this important policy.

HEALTH OF THE NATION – IMPLICATIONS FOR
COUNSELLING

The 1991 Government White Paper *The Health of the Nation* (DoH
1992) selected mental illness as one of five key areas in its health
strategy for the people of England. Targets were also set to improve
mental health in Wales. The primary targets of the White Paper
were:

• To improve significantly the health and social functioning of
  mentally ill people
• To reduce the overall suicide rate by at least 15 per cent by the
  year 2000 from 11.0 per 100,000 population in 1990 to no more
  than 9.4
• To reduce the suicide rate of severely mentally ill people by at
  least 33 per cent by the year 2000 (from the lifetime estimate of
  15 per cent in 1990 to no more than 10 per cent).

In addition there are further, more general aims embedded in
these three targets. These are to:

• improve information systems;
• develop comprehensive local services;
• improve diversion from custody;
• increase alternatives to benzodiazepines (minor tranquillizers); and
• introduce preventive mental health strategies in work settings.

The handbook recognizes that mental illness had 'remained a
poor relation' in management priorities resulting in fragmented and

poorly coordinated services. A principal theme for management action is work with other agencies to promote mental health and reduce the stigma attached to mental illness. The Welsh targets are more detailed and put even more emphasis on reducing stigma, reducing the effects of socio-economic factors on mental health and improving quality of life.

The Health of the Nation: Key Area Handbook on Mental Illness (DoH 1993) makes recommendations to health service planners and managers on achieving the targets and improving mental health services. The handbook tends to concentrate on the financial and social costs to the country of mental illness and suicide. MIND's policy paper on the health of the nation (MIND 1993) recognizes the importance of the strategy and values the potential for building up a range of local preventive services but also points out some risks inherent in the targets. The MIND policy emphasizes the need for greater involvement of users of mental health services in its interpretation of the national targets.

The main direction for change in NHS reforms in the 1990s are towards extended primary care and increasing use of day treatments. *The Health of the Nation* (DoH 1992) sets out the need for the development of comprehensive local services embracing collaborative work, staff development and training and a variety of alternative provision ranging from specialist psychiatric intervention to supportive befriending by voluntary agencies. The handbook includes specific recommendations for counselling and psychotherapeutic work to be offered as part of collaborative care.

THE GATEWAY TO TREATMENT

As *The Health of the Nation: Key Area Handbook on Mental Illness* (DoH 1993) points out, mental health problems are a leading cause of illness, distress and disability and contribute significantly to premature death through suicide. Epidemiological studies suggest that between 10–15 per cent of the population have mental health problems at any one time (Mann 1993). The most common presenting issues are anxiety and depression and the majority of people make an initial contact with their general practice.

> Fortunately we are blessed in the UK in having a comprehensive system of primary care that, despite some fraying at the edges, is still the envy of the world. General Practitioners and their colleagues in the primary health services are the gate-

keepers to all of the services including the mental health ones, even if there is some argument over what exactly constitutes a mental health problem.

(Tyrer, Higgs and Strathdee 1993:xiii)

Psychiatric disorders rank third most common after respiratory and cardiovascular complaints. Strathdee and Sutherby (1993) have summarized the principal research findings into the extent of mental health problems being dealt with in the primary care sector and conclude that up to a quarter of all consultation to an average GP's daily surgeries have a significant mental health component and just under half of these problems are recognized by the doctors. Tylee *et al.* found that 'patients with serious physical disease were five times more likely not to be recognized as depressed than those without physical disease' (1993:327). A common cause of misdiagnosis is where there is a clustering of both mental and physical symptoms. This may be one reason why the elderly are underrepresented in the age profile of mental health statistics. The majority of people diagnosed mentally ill are between 22–55 years. There is also a sex bias in presentation and diagnosis of psychiatric disorders with a ratio of 2.5 women for every man. When GPs fail to recognize serious depression, the treatment offered is not always what it could be. Prescribed drugs may be inappropriate and the suitability of counselling and psychotherapy is not always recognized. To counteract this, the Royal College of General Practitioners set up a fellowship in April 1992 for three years, funded by the Department of Health, Mental Health Foundation and the Gatsby Foundation. Dr Andre Tylee, senior mental health education fellow was appointed to coordinate a national strategy for continuing education in mental health for general practitioners. This includes dissemination of good practice to teach doctors interviewing skills in the context of a ten minute consultation in order to improve their early recognition of depression and anxiety, the risk of suicide and any other primary care needs. General practitioners will also receive training to enable them to develop and deploy their primary care team more efficiently and to widen treatment for depression and anxiety to include social support, counselling and behavioural management techniques, in addition to the use of anti-depressants. Dr Tylee has established a new national cascade structure with the help of the Regional Adviser network, so that eleven regional mental health education fellows have been appointed to train and support the nation's GP tutors and course organizers who teach the GPs and GP trainees. Educational material is being developed for dissemination on schizophrenia, alcohol, and depression in childhood and old age. The Unit for Mental Health Education in Primary Care at St George's Hospital Medical School, University of London, has since been awarded further funding from the Sainsbury Centre for Mental Health to continue the work. The counselling role of general practitioners is explored more fully in the next chapter.

There is promise in the increasing liaison between psychiatry and primary care and the adoption of multi-disciplinary teams, although as we shall see in Chapter 5, this is not yet established across the country. The importance of primary care provision in psychiatric treatment is shown by studies demonstrating that ten times the number of people with all kinds of psychiatric disorder attend primary care services than are referred to psychiatrists (Goldberg and Huxley 1992). About one in four of all psychiatrists has regular clinical contact with primary care services (Tyrer, Higgs and Strathdee 1993). The contribution of Community Psychiatric Nurses, district and practice nurses, occupational therapists, physiotherapists, health visitors, social workers, psychologists and counsellors is further focusing attention on ways of working that can complement medical treatment. Voluntary organizations such as MIND and the National Schizophrenia Fellowship make important contributions to care and act as pressure groups to raise awareness and understanding of mental health issues and to bring about change in policy and practice at local and national levels.

There is a commonly expressed view that the disorders dealt with in primary care are not as serious as those seen by psychiatrists. This is a minimilization of the presenting issues as being not really important, not real mental illness but minor psycho-social problems from which people spontaneously recover. Psychiatrists do come into contact with the most serious of mental disorders but not all of the people with serious mental disorders come into contact with psychiatrists, which may give them a skewed view of their workload and an underestimation of work increasingly being done by counsellors in general practice and the voluntary and independent sectors.

THE COSTS OF MENTAL ILLNESS

The massive costs of medications prescribed for mental disorders in primary care, together with costs associated with absence through sickness (certified and uncertified), and early retirements on health grounds are estimated at a staggering £6,000 million (Mann 1993).

This total does not take account of the personal costs to individuals and their families when someone, as in the following example, is labelled mentally ill:

> If people were listened to and offered talking treatments without all the baggage of psychiatric diagnosis and treatment they would never get caught up in the system that creates chronic mental patients. If choices and information were available, some people who have been enormously damaged and twisted by the world would choose the kind of work and exploration that therapy offers, and would be helped and comforted by it. People should be allowed that choice.
>
> > (Wood 1993, quoting from a letter to MIND from a woman diagnosed mentally ill)

Critics of the medico-pharmacological approach (Healy 1990; Breggin 1993) question the meaning and existence of mental illness that can be treated with drugs. This is not just an intellectual dilemma. There are extremely powerful financial stakeholders involved. Evaluations of the effectiveness of counselling in primary care in significantly reducing the cost of inpatient services and prescriptions for drugs are being matched against evaluations of the effectiveness of new psychotropic compounds, which benefit from the huge research budgets of the major drug companies. We can only speculate at present as to whether increased counselling provision in medical settings would reduce the amount of drugs being prescribed. The evidence from the Marylebone Health Centre (see p. 65) indicates that a substantial reduction in the budget for drugs is possible when alternative provision is available.

PSYCHIC PAIN AND PHYSICAL SYMPTOMS

The facts and figures of epidemiological studies and government strategies and policies both conceal and reveal the suffering and pain of individuals. The size of the problem does not detract from the stigma attached to mental illness. Perhaps the knowledge and fear that any of us might suffer in this way during our lives maintains the rejection and contempt, both conscious and unconscious, which can be observed in provision for people with mental illness and handicap (Waitman and Conboy Hill 1992).

This also helps to explain why it is necessary for people to both conceal and reveal their psychic pain in physical symptoms, an issue frequently encountered by counsellors in medical settings.

Counsellors need to understand the complexities of physiological presentation masking, or speaking for, psychological or relationship difficulties. Ella Sharpe (1940) and Joyce McDougal (1986; 1989) both use the idea of metaphors through which the body speaks. Hobson's (1985) vignette of his patient feeling the pain of an empty heart illustrates his belief that metaphors about the human body convey the deepest levels of experience, not just psychosomatic illnesses but every kind of emotional disturbance. By thinking about something in terms of something else it becomes possible to think and experience what otherwise must be denied. And sometimes the body speaks for us. The feelings expressed through our bodies are our first syntax. Feelings directly experienced and physically expressed can be most clearly observed in babies and young children. When William (18 months) meets his friend Yasmin (16 months) their bodies quiver with excitement and their faces shine with eager anticipation. Much the same effect can be observed when lovers meet, although as adults we have generally learned to control and conceal our outward physical signals from all but the most perceptive observers of non-verbal communication. If we are fortunate those feelings are recognized and then translated into appropriate actions and words that are able to contain and integrate powerful and often overwhelming experiences into a language that can be shared with others. Less fortunate and we will know little of that experience and be unable to express our feelings in a way that enables us to transform our experiences. Then our bodies can become our dictionary, our physical symptoms our vocabulary. What we are not able to communicate in language we can express through our bodies.

What we cannot satisfy through a dialogue – with ourselves or with another we must try to satisfy through another medium – another form of expression, which may be just as eloquent. Some alternative forms of expression are positive. They can be creative, life-enhancing outpourings of art, music, literature or gardening. More negative and destructive are the in-pourings. Endless cravings for satisfaction and relief from unnameable needs and longings that can only temporarily be met by food, drugs, alcohol, cigarettes and medicines. As Oscar Wilde said in *The Picture of Dorian Gray*, 'A cigarette is the perfect type of a perfect pleasure. It is exquisite and it leaves one unsatisfied. What more can one want?'.

According to Bridges and Goldberg (1985) the group of people who express their emotional difficulties as somatic complaints is one which is most frequently encountered in primary care. Since they are, at least initially, convinced that their problems are physical and not psychological, referral to mental health professionals are strongly resisted. Counselling within a general practice can act as a bridging process for these clients and others who need to come to terms with psychic pain physically expressed.

Strong user support for this view is to be found in Geraldine Petterson's (1992) qualitative study of user views of counselling in the Forest Hill Road group practice and from voluntary agencies like MIND. Petterson's study was part of a London-wide research project carried out by the London Research Centre for the King's Fund Commission on the future of acute health services in London. It complemented the work of two other studies commissioned by the Kings Fund Centre, the Greater London Association of Community Health Councils' report on London's acute health services from a user perspective and an opinion survey carried out by the Office of Population Censuses and Surveys. An earlier interim report for the King's Fund Commission (January 1992) had already identified the importance of counselling and shown that it was wanted by consumers as an integral part of the health service.

RECOGNITION OF COUNSELLING NEEDS

In Petterson's survey the users of a counselling service in a general practice strongly supported the provision as an appropriate response to their needs. The users at Forest Hill Road had a characteristic variety of prior experiences which brought them to the counselling service. Some had experienced a recent traumatic event such as theft or injury in an assault and needed medical treatment which led to a request for counselling. Others had experienced an acute episode or particular crisis within the context of a long-term dependency on prescribed drugs for depression. Experience in hospitals had so distressed and disturbed some of the participants, that they sought counselling as a means of coming to terms with both the information they had been given and the state of shock they felt at being given it in an abrupt, sudden and matter of fact manner. These kinds of experiences are frequently suffered by patients already frightened by the unfamiliar environment of a hospital setting. Hardened professionals fail to appreciate their impact often defending themselves from the patients' trauma, stress and pain. Kübler-Ross (1989) recalls that patients told of a fatal diagnosis without a sense of hope had the worst reactions and never reconciled themselves to the person who broke the news so cruelly. This is clear from their accounts of being given bad news:

There is no good way of telling a parent that his or her child is handicapped but there are some which are bad or even worse . . . these should be avoided. In my case the paediatrician stood by my bed – he didn't even fully close the curtains so everyone outside could hear. He just said that my son had Down's syndrome and then left before I could say anything. He hadn't even bothered to wait till my husband returned.

(Ditchfield 1992:19)

I was originally told by a consultant psychiatrist to surround myself with cotton wool and accept the fact that I would be unable to work again.

(Male user of the mental health service in letter to MIND, Woods 1993:16)

At the end of the session he said (to my daughter) 'what shall we put down for Mummy's next appointment, shall we say Mummy's du-lally' he then laughed.

(Account of abuse sent to MIND, Woods 1993:22)

Clearly there are implications for continuing staff development and collaboration with other professionals, a theme that will be developed in Chapter 5. Counsellors faced with this kind of feedback concerning co-professionals have to deal with their own anger, outrage and helplessness at such crassness and cruelty. Many patients have a high regard for much of their medical care but the effect of the illness on the individual is not always adequately recognized. Counsellors in medical settings work with the psychological impact that illness has on the individual. Illness is often extremely traumatic and has enormous implications for the patients' life both in everyday practical terms and in deeply emotional ways. Patients are faced with thoughts, fears and situations they could not possibly have envisaged. This is particularly hard for them in hospital settings where there is often no time available for medical staff to build up a trusting relationship which encourages exploration and self-disclosure. However, when there is access to counselling services the distress and anxiety can be responded to appropriately.

DEALING WITH THE MEANING OF ILLNESS

This very particular role of counselling in medical settings is vividly encapsulated by the perhaps unlikely example from the world of a very small child. Samuel, aged 2½ years, has a 'pocket coat'. However often his mother refers to it as his 'coat pocket' he knows that for him it is too significant for the words to take her order of priority. For this is where Samuel keeps all his bits and pieces, his most secret, prized and precious possessions. The counselling space in medical settings needs to be a pocket coat. If medical treatments strip us painfully bare, physically and emotionally, we need a place and time to make some personal meaning of our experiences if we are to transform them in a way that makes it possible for them to be integrated and tolerated within the whole of our experience. This leads us to examine the relationship between mind and body, body and mind, and the meaning of illness.

Groddeck (1977), writing on the meaning of illness concluded that adults, unlike children, do not understand symbolism easily, and only occasionally grasp symbolic connections. He believed that illnesses expressed a striving of the unconscious to speak a message through an alternative medium. Nina gives us an example of what Groddeck meant: Nina's brother was killed in a road traffic accident and she was called to identify his body. This was naturally upsetting for her but she coped well and put on a brave face. Some time afterwards Nina visited her doctor to complain of severe pains in her face, especially in her nose. The GP was a sensitive woman who had concerns about prescribing the painkillers that Nina requested, and suggested that she talk to the practice counsellor.

Nina began to talk about her brother's death and her experiences of identifying him. He had suffered severe facial injuries and his nose had been completely skewed to one side. As she spoke Nina linked this to the excruciating pain in her own nose and then said, 'I am feeling his hurt in my body.' Unable to face her distress her face had distressed her. Once she was able to talk about her psychic pain Nina stopped feeling it physically.

If we cannot say, or perhaps more accurately know, that we are upset, hurt and angry, that we feel bewildered and crushed by our experience, that we are stressed by overwork or feel alone and unsupported, then living in that experience may be all that is available, as it was for Charlie. Charlie nursed his wife throughout the last year of her life. A strong, healthy man of 58, Charlie never complained or expressed resentment. A month after his wife's death, Charlie felt severe chest pains and feared that he was having a heart attack. Extensive investigations showed that Charlie's heart was in a physically enviable condition for a man of his age – but it still hurt him. Another month passed and Charlie started to feel such pain in his legs that in his words he 'couldn't stand it'. The pain was especially bad at night when it kept him awake and then he would begin to think about his wife. Again, no physical cause could be found to account for these pains – but they still hurt him. Charlie was extremely resistant to any suggestion that he might be hurt by the loss of his wife. Unable to admit emotional pain, Charlie continues to hurt in various parts of his body.

Illness is, as Susan Sontag (1978) says, the night side of life, a more onerous citizenship. We might frame it in an illness or become imprisoned in the psyche to allow the only kind of freedom that makes existence possible, with no parole for good behaviour. 'Psychic prisoners' cannot recognize their own feelings or reflect on the meaning of relationships. They are unable to play out in fantasy different ideas and when the subterranean stream of unconscious life is contacted there can be terrible effects. Maybe the empathy that carers feel for people who suffer in this way is linked to what Balint (1989) describes as the queer mixture of profound suffering and determination that makes them truly appealing. Main describes a more pessimistic syndrome:

> The patients suffer severely and have special needs which worry all around them. They tend to exact strained, insincere goodness from their attendants which leads to further difficulties, to insatiability, to a repetitive pattern of eventually not being wanted and to the trauma of betrayal; it also leads to splits in the social environment which are disastrous for the patient and the continuance of treatment.
>
> Sincerity by all about what can and what cannot be given with goodwill offers a basis for management that, however, leaves untouched the basic psychological problems, which need careful understanding, but it is the only way in which these patients can be provided with a reliable modicum of the kind of love they need, and without which their lives are worthless. More cannot be given or forced from others without disaster for all. It is true that these patients can never have enough.
>
> (Main 1957:144–5)

There are very important implications here for diagnosis and assessment before referrals are made to counsellors and for counsellors in medical settings to be well prepared by their training to consider and assess the suitability of clients for counselling.

McDougal (1986) asks under what conditions it must be possible to build a bridge across the frightening gap that separates psyche and soma – and at what cost to the individual. She concludes that it calls for a particular kind of therapy, what Winnicott (1971) called the 'creative capacity for play'. Markus, Murray Parkes, Tomson and Johnston (1989) describe psychological problems in general practice as the part of their clinical work that most GPs find the most challenging. This is certainly borne out by The Royal College of General Practitioners' need to establish a national programme of education in consultation skills to improve detection of depression and anxiety. There are also important implications for the role of general practitioners to incorporate the counselling skills of listening, observing and understanding the sense that people make of their own situation, helping them to adapt and to find their own solutions. It is also vital that GPs have a good understanding of the counselling process if they are to make realistic referrals to counsellors.

MIND AND BODY

Counselling in medical settings will include a number of clients who present with psychosomatic, somatic and completely fictional disorders in addition to those suffering psychological reactions to a physical illness. Others present with physical and psychological illness as a reaction to, or result of, social and environmental conditions. These are not always easy to separate since emotional states do produce physical changes. When people are generally stressed and anxious, the release of adrenalin can and does cause the heart to pound and the stomach to churn. More account is taken of the physical ailments of clients diagnosed as having psychological problems during counselling in medical settings than in other counselling contexts. Evidence shows that psychiatrists are less likely to detect physical illnesses in women and the elderly (Williams *et al.* 1993). It is as important to recognize the anxiety-producing effects of physical illness and environmentally adverse agents as it is to recognize when there is a primary psychological anxiety (Rippere 1987). The notion that anxiety states are 'all in the mind' is not only dismissive and undermining of an individual's suffering, it is also clinically unsound. A number of organic causes have been identified relating to anxiety states including cardiovascular, pulmonary and endocrinal disorders, and diseases of the nervous system – as the experience of one patient showed. 'I was nearly dead of heart failure with a cupboard full of tranquillisers and sleeping tablets' (User of mental health services, MIND 1993).

The side-effects of drugs and that most common of stimulants, caffeine, can produce or mimic anxiety states, as does withdrawal

from them. Connor (p. 36) emphasized the need to consider environmental and physical factors and to treat and exclude these
appropriately before judgement can be made about the extent of
psychological anxiety. Even when physical and environmental factors are identified and symptoms have abated counselling may still
be needed to adjust to the absence of symptoms, especially if these
have had disabling and chronic effects on a person's lifestyle.

The most important starting point, say the clients, is to be listened
to and respected. In MIND's 'People First' survey, 60 per cent of the
patients who were interviewed found their general practitioner
helpful and 62 per cent that their general practitioner adopted a
positive attitude towards them. 'He discusses alternatives to drug
therapy. He is keen on exercise and natural ways of living, he lets
me go at my own pace.' However, a number of users were concerned
that if they were labelled as having mental health problems that
their physical symptoms would not be taken seriously. 'Just gives
sick notes every twelve months. He wanted to give me an indefinite
note so he wouldn't have to see me again. He doesn't have any
sympathy with mental health problems.' (Rogers and Pilgrim 1993,
quoted in MIND 1993).

FAMILY INFLUENCES

Apart from inheriting genetic predispositions, the health of individuals may be affected by their family systems, their myths, secrets,
taboos, and denials which determine their repertoire of available
behaviour to deal with their experiences. Robin Skynner and John
Cleese (1983) have done much to popularize these ideas in *Families
and How to Survive Them*. When members of a family are prohibited
from expressing their individual thoughts and feelings they have to
find alternative forms of expression:

> A family where people tend to speak for each other and share
> not only the same ideas but also emotions and bath towels, the
> 'enmeshed family' may find it harder to quarrel and express
> themselves as individuals; they have to repress a lot of thoughts
> and feelings and this leads subsequently to psychological prob-
> lems, particularly psychosomatic disorders.
>
>   (Markus *et al.* 1989:117)

Gena's family was much as Markus describes above. They all
talked a lot to each other but never about their innermost thoughts

and feelings. Gena learned at an early age that the only way to get her mother's attention was to complain about pains in her stomach. In spite of missing a good deal of time at school she got the results she needed for a place at university and accepted it, even though her mother tried to persuade Gena that she was not strong enough to manage on her own. Gena walks the earth as if at any moment she might fall forever. She manages to look very old and very young at the same time. She is very anxious and has experienced a couple of fainting episodes since leaving home. These have brought her to the university's student health service where she has explained to the doctor that her pulse is too fast. Gena is studying biology and is concerned that she now has a major heart disorder as well as severe abdominal pains. The doctor, sensing a heartfelt need for attention suggested that, in addition to her physical examination, Gena could also talk with one of the health service's counsellors, to which she agreed.

Gena and her counsellor agreed to work together for weekly sessions of one hour for the remainder of the academic year and then to review the contract. During these sessions Gena talked so rapidly that she was breathless and exhausted by the end of the hour. It was as if she had to produce an endless stream of words to maintain herself and her counsellor. Breaks in counselling coincided with such acute abdominal pain that Gena was admitted to hospital five times and underwent surgery twice during the following two years. No organic disorder was ever found.

Gena's counsellor had her own ideas about separation anxieties but refrained from direct interpretations, gently pointing out the patterns of behaviour together with the absence of any other vocabulary of feeling. As Gena began to be able to get in touch with emotional aspects of herself that she had previously denied or been unaware of, she became able to talk about her distressing and angry feelings. Gradually Gena was able to tolerate breaks without physically acting out a violent reaction to being cut off and she was able to successfully complete her degree course and move away from her parents to begin an independent life.

This is an example of what Freud called *organ speech* used by Cheshire *et al.* (1987) to explain why children suffering recurrent abdominal pain needed to talk with their bodies. And why with this particular part of their body? Their finding was quite specific. The children in their research study had developmentally primitive anxieties about separating from their mothers, but these anxieties were denied within the families. The children were afraid of individuation and of rejecting their mothers. Since any conversation was also out of the question the result was regression to pre-verbal somatization. Where else could this symbolic somatic expression be located but in 'cutting the cord'? As is seen with Gena these symptoms can be taken on through adult life, and appropriate counselling intervention can be deeply effective. But medical practitioners and counsellors need to be aware of these presentations and their meanings if symptoms are to be dealt with rather than reinforced.

There is other evidence that personality types are more prone to certain diseases. For example, those who are ambitious, aggressive, impatient and intolerant, are more likely to suffer a heart attack than those who are more easygoing. It is much more likely, however, that specific diseases are the result of a complex interaction of biopsychosocial factors, and if this is the case, it supports the need for treatments to mirror the causal factors with an interaction of medical, psychological and social services available to clients. Counselling and psychotherapy in medical settings would then be regarded not as a replacement for medical treatment but as necessary and complementary to the healing process.

People who are by nature anxious or who are stressed at work or in their home lives often react with behaviour that leads into a well known but nevertheless vicious circle of anxiety leading to physical symptoms, which increase anxiety. People's anxieties affect the way that they attend to and explain their experiences of pain and illness. The term psychosomatic disorders embraces those physical symptoms, real, detectable and painful enough in themselves, which reflect the psychological state of the client and which can sometimes be detected by linking the way that the physical symptom is described to a feeling state.

Chloe, a nurse who is also a single parent, describes her debilitating stomach condition as a churning sensation that leaves her feeling nauseous. She also says of her colleagues at work, 'I'm sick to death of the way they treat me, but I can't complain because I need the job. It's well paid and I'm frightened that I won't be able to get another one.'

When physical symptoms cannot be linked to any causal explanation or abnormality through medical procedures they might be considered *somatoform disorders*. It is always best to be cautious about the use of this label. There are plenty of examples of *neurotic* somatoform diagnoses which turned out to have a variety of physical causes including tumours, thyroid and other endocrinal disorders, epilepsy and multiple sclerosis. Physical conditions and somatising can coexist as the following example shows.

THE GIRL WHO COULD NOT STOP SNEEZING

In a paper on psychoanalysis in a general hospital setting, Goldie (1986) tells of a dramatic case of intractable and exhausting sneezing, (impossible to simulate), in a 12-year-old girl, which resulted in her admission to hospital for several weeks as an inpatient. Arrangements were made for psychotherapy which proceeded with no direct reference being made to the sneezing; no direct questions asked, and no medical history taken. Previously the girl had been treated as a disease and given no opportunity to express her feelings, and every contact had centred on the physical aspects of sneezing. It emerged during her meeting with the therapist that the girl was living in dread of her family breaking up and that she was powerless to stop it happening. As she began to acknowledge that her 'illness' was a way of preventing her father leaving her and her mother, she was able to get in touch with the sense of loss and sadness beneath her fears and sobbed for a considerable time. After this the sneezing stopped and never recurred.

Goldie's findings support the case for offering counselling and psychotherapy within hospital settings. He suggests that resistance and delay may be due to professional rivalry. When all medical treatments have been exhausted, counselling and psychotherapy cannot alter what is happening but they can offer the possibility of transforming the experience. By allowing time, undivided attention and confidentiality, a dialogue can take place in which there is 'an increase in the density of the communication, (nearer to poetry than banter)' (Goldie 1986:30). This is fundamentally different to any messages that are about reassurance and compliance and highlights the gap between what is often communicated explicitly and implicitly to patients in medical settings.

Explicit	*Implicit*
Try not to think about it	= I can't bear to think about it
Don't you worry yourself	= Don't you worry me
I know just how you feel	= I know just how I feel
Look on the bright side	= Cheer me up
It's not as bad as it might be	= Don't give me a hard time
You'll feel better tomorrow	= Let's not talk about it

Somatization is a complex business. The stigma attached to psychiatric disorders is strong and primitive linkings of mad and bad still persist. Being able to attribute illness on factors outside the self avoids blame, guilt and responsibility. The new demons and spirits that possess us are mystery viruses and toxins. Howard and Wessely

(1993) in their reviews of the psychology of multiple allergy, quote psychosomatic research which suggests that social and cultural factors such as journals, clinics and self-help groups are important in the continuation of people's symptoms and contribute to a feeling of being understood that is lacking when the medical profession fails to acknowledge their suffering. The media also appears to be influential in people's self-diagnosis, which change between multiple chemical sensitivity, total allergy syndrome, chronic fatigue syndrome and food allergies. Evidence shows that patients with total allergy syndrome tend to also have long-standing psychological problems and a history of somatic symptoms.

Counselling is generally regarded as less stigmatizing than referral to psychiatric services and may well be more acceptable to clients suffering psychosomatic and somatoform disorders in addition to those coming to terms with the effects of physical illnesses. The engagement in a counselling relationship with its acceptance of the client's personal meaning and explanation of illness together with appropriate medical treatment can mobilize the person's participation in their own healing, as one grateful client found:

> [Counselling] helps to bring everything together – you can't really separate who you are and the workings of your mind from your body.

> ... it's put me back in charge of my life – that's why it's so important – I'm in control ...
>
> (Petterson 1992:3)

· FIVE ·

Professional relationships in counselling in medical settings

Where do counsellors fit in medical settings? According to the Counselling in Medical Settings Division of BAC one of the most widely expressed concerns of counsellors in medical settings, particularly those in hospitals, is their sense of isolation. The paradox is that they work in the context of a vast web of interdependent professional relationships. Ben's experience illustrates the paradox: he smiled wryly as he said to himself, 'I haven't seen a soul all day.' As a full-time counsellor in a large hospital in the South of England Ben is unusual in that he is not a nurse, nor does he have a background in a medically related field. He works all day with terminally ill patients and their families. What Ben is saying is that he has not seen any of his colleagues, managers, pals, buddies, mates – his own life-support network. He works alone while apparently being surrounded by other caring professionals.

In being theoretically part of a team, while actually not being part of it, Ben does not fit into any of the recognizable, though sometimes hidden, formal though sometimes informal, professional and occupational groupings at the hospital. There is considerable potential in his situation for the expression of envious and territorial disputes to break out between counsellors and medical staff. And when, unlike Ben, the counsellor's job is split between counselling and another primary vocational role, this can apply to inner and outer experiences, causing confusion, ambivalence and dilemmas as we saw in the case of Allie on p. 87.

CARING FOR THE CARERS

Heidi's experience (p. 89) showed that nursing staff were not in-
clined to develop and maintain the support networks they said they
wanted. This is in spite of the emphasis that such support is given
in a publication aimed at raising awareness of health promotion in
medical settings. *Health at Work in the NHS* (HEA 1992) gives initial
information and advice, including ideas for the development of
support networks in the workplace and for links with other people,
organizations and resources already available. These include:

• Fourteen regional Look After Your Heart (LAYH) workplace
  officers
• Local health education/promotion department
• Voluntary networks such as Relate, MIND
• In-house groups – occupational health staff, health and safety,
  staff committees
• Networking and training events, consultative workshops
• Resource packs, policies and guidelines.

This initiative requires that a senior person in the organization be
delegated to deal with the day-to-day issues and act as a coordinator.
This should be a clearly specified part of their job description and
be reflected in their performance objectives. However, to allocate this
role does not automatically resolve the issues, as Mairi discovered.
As she herself said, 'My manager is the *last* person I would talk to
if I had any health or personal problems.' Mairi is a staff welfare
adviser and her concern reveals the hidden agendas related to staff
appraisal and promotion prospects that are concealed behind bland
policy statements and her fears about confidentiality.

We have already seen that there are often real difficulties in
generating interest and involvement in staff support groups. This
initiative will need to attract genuine staff involvement and support
and not be seen as being imposed by management, if it is not to
become a hollow exercise or be limited to effecting changes in safe
and peripheral activities such as cycle storage facilities, sales of to-
bacco products and displays of health promotion posters. Here is an
opportunity to care for staff and change attitudes by providing confidential counselling and support services as the norm rather than
as signals of weakness and failure, thus inhibiting take-up.

The theme of the counsellors' experience of their work setting
reflects a common experience amongst health care staff. The need
for, and the lack of, supportive individual and group opportunities
is identified by Aveline (1992) in a discussion of the training group

component of a multi-disciplinary psychotherapy course for health care professionals, mainly employed in mental health. Aveline states that:

> ... the seeming absence of emotional support in the institutions where members work, points to an unmet need among staff. Members have often expressed their regret at the lack of supportive settings in which difficulties, past and present, could be explored and, furthermore felt that their professional role was incompatible with such expression. To disclose personal problems was to invite the accusation of undesirable weakness from others, and from their rigid, internalised role model which stated that carers have to be strong.
>
> (Aveline 1992:128)

This is certainly borne out by my own experience over the past ten years of facilitating training groups and supervising trainee counsellors from the whole range of medical settings. Even given that people's feelings reflect an interactive mix of inner and outer experiences and that some of the inhibitory fears of persecution and punishment reflect their internal worlds, the frequency and similarity of feelings and experiences expressed point to an outer reality that cannot be ignored. As the following example demonstrates, Joseph unconsciously selects the most apt expression to describe the interplay of his inner and outer experiences.

Joseph feels totally unsupported in his counselling work in an armed forces hospital. His manager wants his work to be invisible, wants him to clear things up as speedily and cleanly as possible. 'How can I talk to her – or any of the others about my feelings?', asks Joseph, 'when we meet in the mess every day; we eat together in the mess, talk together in the mess, we live together in the mess.'

RELATIONSHIPS WITH OTHER PROFESSIONALS

Experiences in training groups reveal, through a parallel process, the relationships that exist within medical settings. They show a scene of occupational rivalry set against a background of hierarchical structures, archaic assumptions and vocational stereotyping. The heightened awareness generated by the group work exaggerates both the interpersonal and social factors that affect all of our communication. Group experiences can enable participants to reflect on how their attitudes and beliefs are transferred from one situation to another, as Mariette discovered.

Mariette insisted that her silence in the group was because there was nothing she wanted to say. Trained initially as an occupational therapist, Mariette had since qualified as a counsellor and saw this as an integral part of her work. In her multi-disciplinary team meetings at work she constantly felt that she had to balance out the needs of the clients, her own thoughts and values, her expertise as a counsellor, and the need to maintain a relationship with the other staff in the team whom she perceived as having higher status but fewer credentials in counselling. Mostly she remained silent. During the training group discussions Mariette realized that she had become so accustomed to defending herself in the territorial conflicts at work that she found it hard to imagine that she could discuss her work without being 'put in her place'. Mariette discovered that she had internalized the unspoken collusive rules of her work team. She did have a choice about what she could think and say but was so constrained by her own perceptions of her role and status at work and by others' behaviour towards her that she had no voice.

Historically determined social interaction in medical settings has set the guidelines for our interpersonal behaviour. Much of this is bound up with age, gender, ethnic origin, education, qualifications and position in the medical hierarchy. Doctors are clever, well-educated and therefore entitled to lead others; nurses are academically limited and therefore entitled to serve others. Neither of these historical stereotypes do justice to reality but are still played out in a Goffmanesque interpretation of the roles, where the rules of engagement are clear to all, even if they are never articulated (Goffman 1961).

In one university health service the hierarchical structures of the personnel are reinforced by the building itself. In this spatial metaphor for the status of the staff the doctors and nursing staff work on the top floor, normally accessed by lift, the counsellors on the floor below and ancillary and support services on the ground floor. There is tension between the expressed policy of coherence and unity within the service and the tendency to fragment into sectional interests. The doctors are remote figures, rarely seen about the building and represented by a nurse at the team meetings. The nurse is frequently late for the meetings, mainly silent, sits separately from the rest of the group, though co-operative on any issues which affect her section. The secure, autonomous professional presence of the doctors allows them to delegate this task. They accept referrals from and make referrals to the counsellors but remain largely invisible, cloaked by the superior demands of their role.

The entrance of a new character in any drama heightens our awareness of existing relationships and raises our curiosity about potential new alliances and conflicts. The introduction of counsellors into medical settings poses questions. What are the rules? Where do these people fit into the existing structures? For staff employed as nurse/counsellors the problem is solved by carrying forward patterns of behaviour from previous experiences, even though these may be inappropriate for the counselling role and give rise to disquiet for Mariette; to the eternal dilemma for Allie (p. 87); and to the denial described by Heidi (p. 89). For staff employed as counsellors the problem determining the rules of engagement may be resolved by linking their appointment to another occupational pay scale or by appointing them on limited-term contracts. Counsellors in university health services might be employed on the lecturer scale; in hospitals on nursing or ancillary staff scales. In primary health care counsellors are employed on an extremely wide variety of contracts and pay scales. Why should counsellors be on lecturer/nurses/secretarial pay scales? These disparities reveal as much about the employers' and managers' understanding and attitudes towards counselling as they do about confusion over the content of the role and the different levels of training and qualification for counselling. There is an urgent need to review this and determine counselling pay scales by building on the very good work begun by the BAC's *Guidelines for the Employment of Counsellors in General Practice* (BAC 1993b) and in FHSAs such as Derbyshire where the three elements of management, vision, administration and leadership have combined to produce a coherent scheme for the employment of counsellors in general practice (Derbyshire FHSA 1994).

Managers at best combine vision, administrative skills and leadership and need to be very clear about where and how counselling roles fit into their whole care strategy, otherwise, and this would explain the sense of isolation felt by many counsellors in hospitals, there is a danger that it will become marginalized, misunderstood and misrepresented. Then it will inevitably be a low priority area, often not even included within the organizational structure as an ongoing service. If managers do not understand counselling – do not even know if their staff are qualified (see p. 43) – or what they would be qualified in if they were; or what counts as a 'proper' qualification; or why they need supervision which takes place during working hours, it is not surprising that they sometimes misuse their trained and competent counsellors. If managers do not understand what being qualified as a counsellor means, they may well think that a two-day training course is sufficient, because 'we're all counsellors in medical settings'. The oldest cliché still reverberates in Francis' ears.

Francis was appointed to set up a counselling and information unit in a specialist hospital department. Full of energy and enthusiasm he began to conduct assessment interviews for the many referrals he received from social workers and consultants. Because he had no medical background or training he understood little of the hierarchies and rules of behaviour in the hospital and found it increasingly difficult to make alliances with other staff. Referrals began to be erratic. Not only were inappropriate referrals made from within his own department, Francis started to receive clients from all the other hospital departments. Francis' struggle to be recognized as a professional was seriously affected by these pressures as was the ongoing evaluation of his work.

All of Francis' attempts to collaborate with the medical staff were thwarted and he was criticized for setting standards too high, for example, on the need for confidentiality and time to assess clients' suitability for counselling. Clearly Francis' version of counselling and his attitudes and beliefs about his role did not match his colleagues' expectations. The question of what others expect from counsellors and how the counselling role fits into the medical hierarchy and value system has great relevance for its incorporation as a distinct healing process within a health service that is increasingly charged with the management of collaborative health care.

COLLABORATIVE CARE

A common theme throughout the major NHS initiatives for the 1990s is the need for collaborative care systems that will meet individual needs in the community. Given the disparate nature of multi-disciplinary teams within several contexts, each having to define their own ways of working together in times of change, this constitutes an enormous co-operative venture. In this chapter we look at the way that counselling fits into the vision of collaborative care at the national policy level, through *The Health of the Nation* (DoH 1992) and at the management of counselling through care in the community. This will lead us to looking more closely at the counsellor's role and professional relationships across a range of health care provision as examples of the vision and its management and administration in practice.

What is the glue that can hold this collaborative venture together?

There has to be a strategy that can establish common values, beliefs and attitudes towards health care, and a coherent vision, if there is to be any coherence and cooperation. As we saw in Chapter 4, national health promotion strategies such as *The Health of the Nation* (DoH 1992) set out policies with explicit statements of intent with measurable targets for health gain. *The Health of the Nation: Key Area Handbook on Mental Illness* (DoH 1993) for promoting mental health clearly identifies the need for counselling and psychotherapy. In England and Wales managers and planners have been charged with the duty of improving mental health services:

> Significant opportunities now exist for the effective treatment and continuing care of people with acute and severe and enduring mental illness and the reduction of suicide rates. Developments include changes in treatment methods – particularly the development of psychotherapies, including cognitive, behavioural, interpersonal and family therapies . . .
>
> (para 1.6:12)

A major area of direct health promotion work is the detection of at-risk groups and the *provision of advice and counselling*, for example in connection with

- disemployment [*sic*] – redundancy and retirement;
- family formation – genetic risks, environmental hazards, avoidance of drugs, nicotine and alcohol;
- family circumstance – bereavement, single parenting, befriending
- social isolation;
- living conditions – homelessness;
- sensory/physical impairment – to reduce risk of depression;
- child abuse – early detection and management;
- awareness of mental health – stress management and self care.

(para 2.5:28)

The Health of the Nation: Key Area Handbook on Mental Illness takes a broad view of the provision that will be needed to pursue targets of reducing the numbers of suicide and improving people's 'social functioning'. The handbook recommends building alliances in a 'much broader area than that set by health and social services provision' (DoH 1993, para 2.10:30). It suggests joint working arrangements with voluntary and statutory organizations. This offers an increased opportunity for access to counselling from a range of previously unco-ordinated sources and a higher profile for counsellors as partners in the alliance.

INTERAGENCY COLLABORATION

In his gloomy prognosis of the collaboration between local authority services and voluntary bodies, Tyndall (1993) foresees not equal
partnerships but increasing pressures on the voluntary bodies to
become the social services privatized sector. Drawing on the evidence of caseworkers from the Tavistock Institute, Tyndall reports on
a three-year interdisciplinary study programme with voluntary marriage guidance counsellors, general practitioners, social workers,
probation officers and health visitors. This study revealed the difficulties of collaborative work, as using the structures and boundaries
of the different agencies was used as a defence rather than as an
opportunity for cooperation.

This reminds me of a well known simulation exercise which I
have used on several occasions at multi-disciplinary and inter-agency
staff training events. The exercise requires competing teams to find
individual and/or whole group solutions in a save the human race
scenario, working against the clock. The only successful outcome
possible is for *all* of the teams to collaborate in finding the solution.
A repeated and salutary outcome is that in the majority of cases the
teams opt for solutions that lead to the destruction of everyone
rather than make alliances that offer salvation.

The salutary outcome of the study noted by Tyndall is that the
group members least able to form collaborative relationships were
the counsellors. Confidentiality was usually given as the reason for
not working together but the validity of this was not tested. Counsellors in medical settings frequently complain about feeling isolated, but this study poses some interesting questions about the
nature of counselling relationships, their privacy, even secrecy and
the nature of people who become counsellors, people who perhaps
prefer not to work with others. Counsellors like Ben, (see p. 107)
feel the disadvantages of working alone but also value the advantages, 'I like my autonomy and not having somebody checking
what I do, I like the safe intimacy.' It is this autonomy, this safe
intimacy that can arouse envy in other staff who cannot understand the need for private counselling space and time for the client
and see it as a luxury for the counsellor, compared with their own
stressful working conditions.

Tyndall's conclusion is not ultimately pessimistic. Collaborative care
is possible if all the partners are fully confident about their own
work, and understand and trust each others' contributions. When
this is the case referrals can be made honestly and appropriately, in
the best interests of the client. When the network is characterized

by lack of information and understanding, there is a danger that referrals might be used as a means of solving the referrer's problem rather than offering a genuine opportunity for help. Francis' experiences (see p. 12) are an example of this but there are also examples of good practice. Connor's work in the substance misuse clinic (see p. 36) takes place in a setting that is characterized by harmonious internal and external relationships and teamwork. Referrals are made to this specialist unit from general practice, social services, probation and prison services and hospitals. Judgement is exercised within the substance misuse team on issues such as whether or not to accept referrals. Treatment protocols and staff autonomy and expertise are respected by the other agencies and by the Consultant Psychiatrist who has ultimate clinical and medical responsibility for clients. Connor is clear that being confident about his role and the theoretical approach enables him to work independently and collaboratively with general practitioners and psychiatrists, who in turn respect his advice and guidance.

CARE IN THE COMMUNITY

If a shared vision is the glue that can hold broad alliances together, internal conflicts within medical settings can dissolve cooperative bridge building activities and obstruct delivery of services. The break up of old alliances with redistribution of resources and consequent shifts in status and power may result in energy being invested in competition, rivalry and spoiling rather than healthy co-operation and collaboration. It is difficult to imagine the needs of the clients taking precedence if they become the piggy in the middle of competing services.

The Community Care Act of 1990 was a major step taken with the intention of liberalizing the psychiatric services in Britain. It determined the closure of large mental hospitals and the release of many people previously labelled *mentally ill* into the community. For about 40 years the question of whether a person's psychological or mental condition can be appropriately included in a medical model of disease has been one aspect of an ongoing and lively debate which has contributed to the current reforms.

Donald Winnicott concurred with his friend John Rickman's definition: 'Mental illness consists in not being able to find anyone who can stand you' (Winnicott 1990:218). R.D. Laing (1967) challenged traditional explanations of schizophrenia and used the term *broken-hearted*. In the United States Thomas Szaz (1974) called mental illness a myth and traced the developments in psychiatry, psychoanalysis and psychosomatic medicine back to a historical paradigm – an over compensation by Charcot, used to secure legitimacy for his case that hysteria should be recognized as a disease by the French Academy. Szaz's work was influential in persuading politicians in the United States that large psychiatric hospitals should be closed. The debate continues and the same evidence and arguments are used by both the political right and left to support their particular views on provision, and by psychiatrists and psychotherapists to support their particular views on treatments.

1 April 1993 was the starting date of this country's community care reforms, a 'snapshot' date to mark the official start of a programme that had been gathering momentum since the 1960s. The ideas may have been around for a long time but the implementation was hasty. In between the Audit Commission's report *Making a Reality of Community Care* (Audit Commission 1986) and the Griffiths Report (1988) the agenda was set in the Act of 1990 to prepare within three years for the challenge of coordinating care between different providers for the whole range of mental health needs within the community.

The aims of community care to close the stigmatizing, depersonalizing and depowering mental hospitals and discharge patients to the care of the community are admirable. The problem is to establish care systems in the community capable of matching the vision and to identify key stakeholders who can implement, direct and evaluate appropriate provision. Teamwork, even within small, closely knit teams can be difficult. How much more challenging to devise and successfully maintain the communication channels and extended teamwork of the Care in the Community Programme.

Dismantling the system has been achieved with impressive speed by the programme of closure of large psychiatric hospitals. However, increased ecological awareness shows us how precarious is the balance between destruction and creation. Short-term measures, which stick a finger in the dike holding back an ocean of needs, will only be sufficient if they are used to give time to prepare for adequate holding and containment. If the only action is to force more fingers into the increasing number of holes, less hands are available to complete more radical constructive work, and none can afford to take their eyes and minds off the impending collapse of the structure.

A patient on a life support machine that is too expensive, outdated, large and cumbersome and needing too much maintenance, needs the transfer to a more efficient and effective machine to be seamless. Switching off the major supply of psychiatric care needed to be accompanied by sufficient funding through the local health authorities for a viable and comprehensive alternative provision, which was adequate to meet the needs of both those discharged as the hospitals closed and of the general population (see Chapter 4). The challenge of juggling new and increased demands on health care systems with budget controls, is likely to continue as the numbers of elderly people grow and advances in medical technology continue. Small acute care units have been established within general hospitals to deal with assessment and emergencies for short-term treatment, but there is still a need for long-stay residential accommodation and supervised care which is catered for by private or health authority provision. Some users stay in acute psychiatric wards for months because there is no supported housing for them. Studies in two acute hospitals found a third to one-half of the patients on psychiatric wards were homeless (MIND 1993). For these patients the question is not only what care, but also what community?

It appears that competition for community health care resources is so fierce that there has to be a tragedy and/or a national inquiry to divert funds into unglamorous services. Additional funding was allocated to the Care in the Community Programme following the Clunis case in 1993 (see p. 127). Reviewing the experience of a client of the care management provided by integrated multi-disciplinary teams (teams of psychologists, psychiatrists, community psychiatric nurses, occupational therapists and psychiatric social workers) Groves (1993) discovered that in Northern Ireland, Scotland and Wales, health and social services systems are better integrated than in England. In England, in spite of the direction from government strategy and policy on multi-disciplinary provision there is apparently a lack of involvement, interest and experience among health professionals, especially the general practitioners, in designing their local systems. In some areas there are still no teams in place to deal with the demands of care in the community. Since, as has already been noted, there are ten times as many people with mental health problems seen in primary care than by the specialist services, the need for interdisciplinary collaboration in provision and training is crucial, not just between general practitioners and psychiatrists but also between team members. When links and networks are in place there can be a high level of satisfaction reported by general practitioners (see p. 121), but general practice is the gatekeeper of mental health, not the safety net.

THE CARE-PROGRAMME APPROACH

This new system is based on a *needs-led* approach to provision and depends initially on the quality of the relationship between local authority Social Service Departments, who both assess needs and provide care, and other partners including the local health authority and voluntary and independent providers. The nature of care programmes is determined by local criteria for eligibility and the resources available but all should have the key features of care packages based on a multi-disciplinary assessment of an individual's needs. This includes meeting with individuals to determine with them their care management plans. It also calls for regular reviews of the needs of people already being treated in the community. The need for counselling to be provided as part of these care packages is identified and recognized within the policy statements.

The internal market has shifted purchasing power to general practitioners who, previously dependent on psychiatric services in secondary care, can now buy services from a range of providers, including independent counsellors. They can also employ practice staff (as therapists, counselling psychologists, nurses and counsellors) all of whom could offer counselling or use counselling skills within their primary occupational role. Critics of these new arrangements argue that there is a danger of diverting funds from psychiatric services. This smacks of rivalry and power issues and can lead to a demand for more research into the efficacy of different types of provision but there is often little reference to the views of the users of these services.

EVIDENCE FOR PROVISION OF COUNSELLING SERVICES FROM USERS

MIND's policies on key topics in mental health have been collated in its *Policy Pack* (MIND 1993). Six sections contain a summary of all of MIND's policies and an action sheet for implementing them. These cover empowerment through user involvement; combating discrimination; addressing social needs; developing mental health services; and rights and standards.

In its policy paper on The Health of the Nation MIND (1993) supports the broad alliance strategy and proposes its own targets to achieve improvements in mental health. These include taking users' views into account and building on the existing support networks. Users' views consistently demonstrate that they value being able to choose between talking treatments and/or medication. Users want access to counselling and need more information about a range of complementary therapies.

The National Schizophrenia Fellowship conducted a survey in 1990 to evaluate its members' views on provision of services in the community and discovered that overall they were all viewed as unsatisfactory. Carers expressed a need for counselling but only 1 per cent had access to any. Of the members diagnosed as schizophrenic, 62 per cent felt they needed counselling but only 12 per cent had access to it.

MIND's Policy recommends increased availability of information on all local services and choice from a range of options at every access point to services, including the general practitioner, the social services care manager, and assessment for a care programme. The options should include provision for emotional support through counselling, befriending, self-help support, psychotherapy, cognitive therapy, complementary therapies and specific provision for separate, identifiable needs such as women-only crisis centres and black counselling services. If services are not available this should be recorded and used in audit for future planning.

MIND is concerned that there should be a balancing out of provision from physical treatment, which includes over four million prescriptions for drug treatment and over one hundred thousand treatments of electroconvulsive therapy (ECT), towards talking treatments. Counselling and psychotherapy should be more widely available. The risks and benefits of physical, pharmacological and talking treatments should be made clear so that people can make their own more informed decisions about options. This is assuming that there are options to choose from.

For people to have access to a range of provision, including counselling, their needs must first be recognized. On average general practitioners fail to detect psychological distress in half of the people who present with such symptoms. There is a wide variation in the ability of general practitioners to recognize anxiety and depression (Freeling et al. 1985). When they are good they are very good – as good as consultant psychiatrists – but when they are bad, the accuracy of their diagnoses is no better than chance (Marks, Goldberg and Hillier 1979).

General practitioners find it easier to recognize depression and anxiety if the person is white, unemployed, recently separated or bereaved, middle-aged and a woman who looks depressed. They fail to recognize psychological distress when people are physically ill or present with physical symptoms, when cues are presented late in the consultation, and when the general practitioner is not personally tuned-in to the expression of feelings. Sally's experience bears this out.

SALLY

Although Sally's outward appearance is cool, calm and confident she says:

> My anxiety shows itself in physical symptoms or even illness. When I'm anxious about anything my stomach churns, my palms sweat, my heart thuds and I breathe more quickly. I had a major crisis in my life and lost a lot of weight quickly. I couldn't sleep very well and spent all my time either overexcited or irritated. I was already on sleeping pills but awake all night. I went back to my GP, thin, tense and agitated. He doubled the dose and offered no other help, not even to ask if I had a problem! It took a long time to get myself together again. If only that doctor had known what to do.

Counselling has not traditionally been a common or well understood and available option. Treatment for anxiety and depression has been almost entirely drug based, with minor tranquillizers being prescribed for major depressive disorders and repeat prescriptions being given without regular review and consultation. 'Heartsink', 'revolving door', 'fat-file' are all labels for patients, who, for reasons that must make sense in some context other than the purely physical or medical, make constant demands for attention from their doctors. How might Sally's doctor be helped to recognize what for her was an obvious plea for recognition of her distress? Can such skills be taught, and can doctors learn them?

A three-year mental health initiative by the Royal College of General Practitioners (see p. 93) and the consensus statement between the RCGP and the Royal College of Psychiatrists for the 'Defeat Depression Campaign' (DoH in press) reflect the belief that it is possible to tackle this problem through education, training and raising awareness. It is also recognized that an essential requirement of these initiatives, of *The Health of the Nation* (DoH 1992) and care in the community that this has to be a collaborative effort. During the first year of this initiative, regional mental fellows were appointed to determine the learning needs of GP tutors, course organizers, GPs and their trainees with respect to mental health issues. This group of regional fellows determined the national and regional priorities for mental health training and reviewed educational resources for dissemination. Scepticism about the effectiveness of this 'top-down' model revolves around questions of whether this is the wrong way round and whether enough attention is being paid to user's views.

RELATIONSHIPS BETWEEN PROFESSIONALS IN THE PRIMARY HEALTH CARE TEAM

Some primary health care teams have many links with counsellors and other staff using a range of counselling and psychotherapeutic techniques. The title counsellor may be used to refer to community psychiatric nurses (CPNs), medical/psychiatric social workers and clinical psychologists in addition to practice counsellors, and some psychiatrists are based within primary health care. Sometimes general practitioners themselves act as counsellors in addition to using their interpersonal skills.

Links between the members of the primary health care team will be stronger if it functions as a team and not a collection of unco-ordinated co-workers. Evidence supports the suggestion that general practitioners value and make good use of mental health professionals, particularly counsellors and community psychiatric nurses linked to their practices. Thomas and Corney (1993) reporting on a survey among general practitioners and their links with counsellors, psychiatrists, community psychiatric nurses, clinical psychologists and social workers, found high levels of satisfaction among general practitioners for counselling and CPN services. A clear outcome of this survey was that general practitioners found closer working relationships with mental health staff to be productive and valuable. A similar outcome was reported by Warner, Gater, Jackson and Goldberg (1993) who conducted a three-year study in South Manchester to determine the effects of a new community mental health service on the practice and attitudes of general practitioners. Ten doctors had access to community mental health teams and ten others continued to use hospital services. The doctors with access to community teams showed significantly more satisfaction with their services, particularly with community psychiatric nurses and community social workers. Easier access resulted in these services being given a higher priority by the doctors. Balestrieri *et al.* (1988) in their meta-analysis of specialist mental health treatment in general practice found evidence that treatment was about 10 per cent more effective when there was contact with specialist mental health staff than if the GP alone was involved.

There are important implications here for the need for counsellors, and staff with a significant counselling role such as CPNs, to have good links with general practitioners and for general practitioners to have a clear understanding of their work and how to access it. It appears that doctors' fears and fantasies about erosion of their clinical freedom and autonomy were allayed by the reality of effective cooperation and communication between general practitioners and the specialist support which offered increased opportunities for discussion.

In Chapter 4 the general practitioner's role as gatekeeper was shown as being well recognized. Ninety-eight per cent of the people in Britain are registered with a practice and 60 per cent of them consult their GP at least once a year, 90 per cent in any two-year period. GPs are first in line to detect and assess patients needs, both physical and mental health disorders. Some GPs are excellent diagnosticians. When people present with physical symptoms these are the doctors who detect underlying depression, anxiety and psychological distress. When people present with long-term mental health disorders, these are also the doctors who detect physical disorders, knowing that 45 per cent will have physical morbidity with standard mortality rates significantly higher than that of the general population (Strathdee and Sutherby 1993). More simply, they have good consultation and interviewing skills; show more interest and concern; ask people about their feelings; make more empathic comments and are sensitive to cues. They relate well, and tend to be older, better qualified than average, more sensitive to their own needs and interested in psychiatry (Marks, Goldberg and Hillier 1979). This group of doctors use basic counselling skills in their consultations. These skills can be learned, if the doctor's personality is not too conservative or resistant. They include being able to maintain eye contact, picking up verbal and non-verbal cues, making more facilitating noises, asking questions about the person's home life and spending a little time clarifying the presenting issues. There is less urgency about these consultations, and they are more person-centred. These doctors are not so afraid that if they allow the person to speak without interruption they will be overwhelmed by a never ending stream of information (Blau 1989). This fear probably underlies the findings from American research that, on average, doctors interrupt people 18 seconds into their presentation. Speaking at the Royal Society of Medicine conference 'Mental Health Care in the 90s and Beyond' (January 31, 1994), on 'How GPs improve their skills in detecting and managing mental health problems', Dr Tony Kendrick reported that experiments to find out how long people actually do talk to their doctors if they are not interrupted show that on average it is between one and one-and-a-half minutes.

Linda Gask and her colleagues (1987; 1991) have shown that improvement can and does take place in doctors' ability to recognize psychological distress. Individual and group techniques using Argyle's (1972) social and interpersonal skills training model are effective if doctors are interested in increasing their competence in this area. More recent developments involving the teaching of communication skills in undergraduate programmes and postgraduate training also offer opportunities to increase competence. The ceiling of improvement is likely to be determined by the doctors' personalities and attitudes, which has implications for the selection of students for medical training and vocational guidance on their appropriateness for different aspects of work.

Clearly, some general practitioners are competent and qualified, willing and able to take on this role. Since Michael Balint's combined training and research groups flourished in the 1950–60s, the number has dwindled, but much of the philosophy has been incorporated into vocational training schemes for general practitioners. For those doctors who want to take a holistic approach, and whose personalities are suited to it, counselling and psychotherapeutic work can enable deeper insight and a clearer understanding of the physical, mental and possible psychosomatic aspects of the person's presenting issues. However, time is a great obstacle and adequate time, even for brief focal counselling and psychotherapy, is a fundamental requirement.

General practitioners who decide to take on a counselling role normally see their clients at the end of surgery times, when they can work uninterrupted for 30–60 minute sessions. This imposes a real limitation on the number of people to whom general practitioners can offer counselling, however suitable their personality, especially when additional time also has to be allocated for supervision. Some GPs find it difficult to embrace a counselling role (Rowland *et al.* 1989; Noon 1992), and if they are confronted with role conflict between relating to patient or client, general practitioners may decide that it would be a better use of resources to refer on to specialist support.

COMMUNITY PSYCHIATRIC NURSES (CPNs) IN THE PRIMARY HEALTH CARE TEAM

The Cumberlege Report on Neighbourhood Nursing (DHSS 1986) recommended that CPNs should remain as part of the specialist psychiatric services team, but there is a counter argument for basing them in primary care settings. When CPNs are based in hospitals, 80 per cent of their referrals are from psychiatrists, but this proportion is reversed when they are based in primary care, where the majority of referrals come from general practitioners. The nature of CPN work changes when their working base is changed. CPNs working in primary health care teams have greater autonomy, larger case loads and more involvement with people with neurotic and adjustment disorders than with psychotic disorders. I asked the members of a team of CPNs, who meet regularly in a support group with other colleagues from a community mental health team in the East Midlands, to tell me about the demand for counselling with their clients. Their responses were unequivocal: 'insatiable'; 'the more you do, the more is needed'; 'it's needed at every level, from psychotherapy to support – and for specific issues such as bereavement and sexual abuse'; '80 to 90 per cent of my work is one-to-one therapeutic relationships; I am almost totally involved in counselling'. When asked about their relationships with other providers, these CPNs saw themselves very much as first line provision. They identified links with a range of other providers, including psychotherapy and psychiatric and social services but equally with voluntary agencies. When the doctors in the study conducted by Warner *et al.* (1993) were asked what their priority would be in setting up a team to work with them in primary care, the majority of those who already had access to a mental health team replied that the community psychiatric nurse was essential.

SOCIAL WORKERS IN THE PRIMARY
HEALTH CARE TEAM

Although, as we have seen, there is evidence of the value of linking psychiatric social workers to primary health care, the numbers of social workers in this setting have declined since cutbacks by local authorities in the 1980s. One general practitioner is reported as asking whether social workers still exist (Thomas and Corney 1993:419).

When social workers are based within primary care there are more opportunities for collaboration, cooperation and appropriate referrals. It is more common to find that social workers are centrally based within social services and liaise with practices to take or make referrals and take part in case discussions. This arrangement reduces the chances of cooperative, trusting relationships forming and slows down communication. Social workers can and do make effective contributions to counselling provision within primary health care, particularly in working with people with depression and relationship difficulties. Social workers are more likely to take into account peoples' relationships and living conditions and offer the kind of practical support that MIND surveys and user's views have shown to be beneficial.

This emphasis on practical support may detract general practitioners from using social workers' skills appropriately. With proper liaison social workers can work with the mix of psychological and social problems that people present. The Community Care Act is also affecting the counselling role of social workers, as they become increasingly involved in assessments for care programmes leaving less time for counselling support.

PSYCHOLOGISTS IN PRIMARY CARE

Clinical psychologists may have specialist training in cognitive/ behavioural therapies and are more likely, though by no means exclusively, to work with people presenting with behavioural problems such as eating disorders, phobias, obsessive compulsive disorders and psychosexual problems. A high level of satisfaction has been recorded for the outcome of behavioural and cognitive therapies, especially where the latter is combined with antidepressant therapy. Studies show evidence that there are savings to be made from reduced prescription of psychotropic drugs which could be used to offset the costs of employing clinical psychologists. Psychologists are seen as particularly useful for their educative and consultative function for the general practitioner, for self-help groups and for the voluntary sector (Strathdee and Sutherby 1993).

PSYCHIATRISTS IN PRIMARY CARE

There are a variety of ways that psychiatrists liaise with the primary health care team. The two most common are the *shifted outpatient clinic*, where the psychiatrist is based in general practice and sees people from the immediate catchment area, and the *consultation model*, where the general practitioner maintains a management role and the psychiatrist acts in an assessment and advisory capacity. Less common is the *liaison attachment model*, where the psychiatrist supervises the primary care team staff but does not work with their clients and the *joint consultation* model with the general practitioner or counsellor.

There are many advantages in linking psychiatric assessments and consultation to the primary care setting. The stigma of referral to a psychiatric department is lessened with the benefit of reduced anxiety and fewer non-attenders. Because the communication between general practitioner and psychiatrist in enhanced there is greater collaboration and continuity of care is more likely.

COUNSELLORS IN THE PRIMARY HEALTH CARE TEAM

We have already seen that about one-third of all general practices consider that they have a counsellor working on site. The title counsellor is used most commonly for CPNs, and then for practice counsellors and psychologists. Alarmingly, counsellors may be employed and work in general practice with no training or qualifications in counselling or any other relevant vocational area. General practitioners refer a wide variety of people to practice counsellors, with issues ranging from marital problems to psychiatric illness. It is very unlikely that, however skilled they are, practice counsellors can deal appropriately with the whole of this range and they will inevitably encounter people with problems outside their sphere of competence. Doctors need to properly understand what their practice counsellors can and cannot do, and need to be discriminating in their referrals if they are to gain the greatest benefit from their counselling provision.

For their part counsellors need to be sufficiently experienced and competent to know the extent of their boundary of competence. The BAC *Code of Ethics and Practice for Counsellors* requires that:

B.2.2.17. Counsellors should monitor actively the limitations of their own competence through counselling supervision/consultative support, and by seeking the views of their clients and other counsellors. Counsellors should work within their own known limits.

B.2.2.19. It is an indication of the competence of the counsellors when they recognise their inability to counsel a client or clients and make appropriate referrals.

(BAC 1993a)

And, in order to work effectively and appropriately as a member of a team, the counsellor needs to have a clear understanding of other roles and resources in the practice and wider community.

Counsellors need to establish contact with social services departments, community mental health services and voluntary bodies in
order to have a clear understanding of the nature and range of
alternative provision and of the various counselling approaches on
offer. In addition to clarifying their understanding of the range
of services, counsellors should have a detailed knowledge of the
medical/psychiatric model, including the signs and symptoms of
major psychiatric illnesses and the implications of prescribed
psychotropic medication, even if they themselves do not use this
model. If we are to offer clients choice of treatment it follows that
we should be knowledgeable about what is available. Furthermore
if counsellors are to work cooperatively with co-professionals and
seek their understanding of the counselling role, equality demands
that counsellors learn about alternative provision. This becomes even
more necessary in the context of care in the community. In addition to knowledge of local statutory and voluntary provision, counsellors need to familiarize themselves with the community care policy,
clearly outlined in the Department of Health's *Community Care in the
Next Decade and Beyond* (1989) and *Caring for People: Policy Guidelines*
(1990).

The case of Christopher Clunis, a schizophrenic who stabbed
and killed Jonathon Zito at Finsbury Park Underground station in
December 1992 is one of a number of incidents involving people
left unsupported to fall into lacunae in community care provision
that tragically match their own inability to cope. Care programmes
are of no avail if the stepping stones in them are too far apart or
have been taken away to build a dam further upstream. Even when
the stepping stones are in place they may be too far off the beaten
track or for permit holders only.

The success of care in the community depends on the links between the different agencies and on adequate funding and resourcing.
Community mental health care depends on strong links between
the primary health care team and mental health professionals.
'Without careful planning areas of community health promotion
will be missed as each member of the team leaves it to somebody
else. Thirty years ago Balint described the same situation in medical
care as the "The collusion of anonymity"' (Lawrence 1993:81).

Working as a team member involves the counsellor in the monitoring and evaluation processes of the practice (Pringle 1993). Counsellors without experience of working in an institutional setting
may find audit and evaluation procedures unusual and irksome.
Some confuse issues of confidentiality with the need to evaluate
their own practice and give the feedback needed for working with

a resource framework. Counsellors should record data for the practice audit and develop their own protocol for the counselling service, which gives details on the methods of referral, the system for making appointments and contacting clients and for record keeping.

Bond (1993) presents a detailed and useful summary of the issues around keeping written records. After weighing up the pros and cons he concludes that record keeping is a part of a systematic and professional approach to counselling that our clients deserve. The BAC/CMS Guidelines recognize that keeping notes of counselling sessions is good practice. The notes should be separate from medical notes and kept in a locked drawer to maintain confidentiality. The Access to Health Records Act of 1990 gives people the right of access to health records made by health professionals after November 1991. Although counsellors are not named in the list defining health professional, BAC advises counsellors in medical settings to assume that their clients may have access to their records. Most people are familiar with the idea of medical records but it is still important to discuss with clients what information is recorded and how it is stored within the practice.

In addition to these administrative procedures, counsellors need to constantly evaluate the effectiveness of their work with clients. Regular supervision, in line with the BAC's recommendations (see p. 69) is an important component of this evaluation. In addition counsellors need to think about basic issues such as how their work fits into the aims of the practice. It is not possible to evaluate effectiveness unless there are some agreed outcomes or criteria to measure against. These criteria should be regarded as an opportunity for counsellors to provide objective evidence to demonstrate the relevance and professional quality of their work. Criteria might include quantitative measures relating to workload, number of sessions, referral routes, prescription rates; and qualitative measures to do with attitudes of other members of the team, changes in their sensitivity and awareness to psychosocial problems, clients' attitudes and ratings of effectiveness. Some counsellors carry out routine evaluations a short time after the end of counselling contracts. These can be brief questionnaires designed to fit into quality assurance monitoring, or more specifically, to check counselling skills, for example, the establishment of a therapeutic alliance.

Being a member of the primary health care team offers the counsellor an opportunity to heighten the other team members' awareness and understanding of the counselling process. If, as the evidence shows, many doctors are unaware of the qualifications of the counsellors employed in their practices (see p. 43), there is a need for more educative work to be done. It is likely that this need extends to the whole team. Balancing the tension between developing and valuing individual autonomy and working collaboratively is at the heart of all genuine teamwork. This does not happen without the involvement of all the team members and an understanding of everyone's personal responsibility, as the following excerpt, taken from an account of setting up a counsellor in primary care, shows:

> All of the staff met once a week at lunchtime to discuss our work and we cast the cordon of confidentiality around the whole of this professional group. Trust enabled us to be open about many things (although familiarity helped us to fail to tackle others). But the method was clear. By involving all our staff, including administrative workers who lived locally, the practice was never allowed to stray far from the path of relevance.
>
> (Curran and Higgs 1993:78)

Being involved as a team member enables a counsellor to contribute to the care of many more people than are seen by appointment in the counselling room. The counsellor's presence, formally and informally can sensitize other staff to the emotional aspects of presenting problems, and help them to think about alternative ways of working with people. This does not only apply to clients. Counsellors can, without taking on a formal counselling or supervision role, affect the culture of medical setting enabling the development of a trusting environment and reciprocal support between colleagues.

· SIX ·

A critique of counselling in medical settings

As a result of its rapid, if uneven growth, counselling in medical settings is characterized by complexity, confusion and considerable differences in assumptions and practice. From the evidence presented in earlier chapters it is clear that clients value counselling as a complementary therapy. What is hard to document or record are the incalculable examples of caring practice that are part of the everyday life of all those involved in this context. It is the very extent and range of what could be called counselling contacts, from a listening ear to brief supportive work to long-term therapy, that contributes to the complexity and confusion. While it is misleading and unhelpful to claim that everyone is a counsellor in medical settings there is a need for appropriately used counselling skills to be recognized as part of everyone's competent interpersonal practice. More clarity and coherence is needed to understand how counselling and counselling skills fit into existing services and, crucially, how these two can be differentiated. The question of whether counselling can develop in medical settings as a separate, yet integrated, service is clearly both central and crucial and it remains to be seen whether it will be incorporated or excluded. The issues affecting that decision include not only strategic policy decisions and cost/benefit analysis but also issues of training, registration, access and equality.

To acknowledge these issues and their implications for implementing counselling into medical settings should not make either the counsellor, the client or the provider so overwhelmingly grateful for *any* provision that they cannot be critical about the appropriateness of referrals. The most appropriate counselling takes place when everyone is clear what is on offer, and what is on offer has been freely chosen by providers and by consumers. But this is often influenced by counselling meaning different things to different people. Breakwell (1987) found in her mapping exercise that nurses in hospitals generally had an understanding of the counselling process and offered non-directive counselling whereas doctors and personnel staff saw counselling as giving advice and problem solving. Such differences can lead to very disparate interpretations of counselling. Without an agreed and shared view of the nature and purpose of counselling provision in medical settings, counsellors can have unrealistic expectations imposed upon them. Parry (1994), appeals for a greater exchange and application of relevant evidence and information from research into counselling in medical settings, deploring the situation, for example, in which many part-time primary care counsellors still find themselves. Often unsupported, having little contact with more specialist services, and without the benefit of an informed decision, some counsellors are being referred the most challenging of clients.

Counsellors who are still concerned and preoccupied with the problems of establishing themselves within medical settings may not want the risk of lobbying those with high status and power to demand a shared involvement in care. However, if counsellors want their service accepted and valued as a healing process in its own right, and to be paid accordingly they have to justify what they do and why it is worth valuing and rewarding. Counselling has to be brought into the open, beyond the safety of the counselling room. Counsellors must walk the tightrope of being collaborative and communicative rather than silent and private, while rigorously maintaining the overriding ethic of confidentiality for their clients. This will not suit people who chose to be counsellors because they prefer to work alone. It may not be easy, but it is essential. Counsellors may have to challenge comfortably held traditions that confuse confidentiality with an unwillingness to openly and honestly explore, examine and evaluate their practice. As counselling is increasingly put under the spotlight by its critics and detractors, counsellors must be ready for the searching scrutiny that follows.

There will also be difficulties in collaboration if there are rigid hierarchical structures within general practices, hospital wards and multidisciplinary teams which create feelings of 'them and us, staff and patient, helper and helped, separated by a great gulf of difference' (Aveline 1992:130). As with all professional carers, the care given can reflect the counsellor's own needs: they really wish to receive what they give. At its worst this can be an abuse of power in which the counsellor fends off personal anxieties by projecting them into others. Florence Nightingale's cautionary words, 'First do no harm', adapted from Hippocrates' famous advice is as useful for counsellors today as it was for nurses in the Crimean War. Guggenbuhl-Craig's (1979) work with carers revealed to him the 'power-shadow', a concealed lust for power, which actually prevents clients making good progress because the carer can only remain powerful if clients fail. These ideas link with Masson's (1989) critique of psychotherapy in which he cites numerous examples of dubious practice to support his accusation that psychotherapy is manipulative and corrupt. However, Masson's claim is the equivalent of accusing the whole of medicine or teaching of immorality because of some instances of abuse. There is an important difference in that these two professions have clear mechanisms for training, registration and disciplinary procedures. Masson's argument and users' evidence (Wood 1993; MIND 1993) all lend weight to the demand for counsellors to be registered and for a national registration body to operate a complaints and disciplinary procedure. This would allow for counsellors and therapists to be struck off and barred from future practice if they contravened recognized codes of ethics and practice.

TRAINING, QUALIFICATIONS AND REGISTRATION

> I think I was really ready to work: all I needed was someone who could stay with me and be untroubled by my trouble. Mary was not that person and while it would be easy to let the kind, well-meaning Marys of this world off the hook, I really think that selection and training, even for voluntary counselling should do better.
>
> (Allen, 1989 quoted in Wood 1993:27)

This client's experience emphasizes the urgent need for counsellors to be appropriately trained and qualified. Many of the major organizational and administrative problems of integrating counselling into general practice have been given direction by the publication of guidelines from the Counselling in Medical Settings Division of BAC. These guidelines provide a useful model for the employment of counsellors in all medical settings but there is a need for further work to produce guidelines for counselling in hospital settings and in interdisciplinary teams. The lengthy and persistent endeavours of the subcommittee within the Counselling in Medical Settings Division to conduct this developmental work must reflect to some extent the difficulties of establishing counselling itself in hospitals.

Valuable as these guidelines are, real advances in establishing counselling as a therapeutic intervention in its own right will not take place until there are more unified and systematic training, accreditation and registration procedures in place. Counselling does not, as yet, have a statutory body to direct its training, qualification and registration procedures. There is growing pressure from voluntary bodies, the media and the professional bodies within counselling and psychotherapy (BAC, BPS, United Kingdom Council for Psychotherapy (UKCP)) to regulate the situation and it is anticipated that a voluntary register will begin in 1994/5. This is, in part, stimulated by the context of European Community (EC) regulations, which would allow counsellors from EC countries where there is a national register to practise in the UK and conversely, prevent counsellors and psychotherapists from the UK who are not registered from practising in other EC countries. BAC's consultative document on a proposal for a National Counselling Register states: 'The power broking between interested parties which is the context in which EC regulations are framed in Brussels is one which favours those who can voice views and needs through national bodies such as government recognised National Registers' (BAC 1992). The professional register envisaged by BAC would involve setting up a register of accredited members who could all demonstrate required standards of competence and who complied with a code of ethics and practice, and which would operate a complaints procedure backed by the kind of sanctions advocated by MIND (Wood 1993:28).

The major professional bodies are all moving towards regulation but are at different stages. The British Psychological Society (BPS) already has Government recognized chartered status which requires a statutory registration. Charter status restricts the use of a particular title. The title Chartered Psychologist is restricted to people who have completed a six-year training made up of a three-year undergraduate degree in psychology and three subsequent years of postgraduate professional training and supervision, with adherence to a code of conduct. The United Kingdom Council for Psychotherapy launched its register in the House of Lords in 1994, the first step towards psychotherapy becoming recognized as a profession, accessible, accountable and authoritative, in preparation for acceptance in Europe. Foundation work conducted by the NCVQ on setting standards of competence for staff employed in advice, guidance, counselling and psychotherapy is contributing towards the development of a comprehensive qualification structure. There is also an expansion of provision of counselling and psychotherapy training in higher education. New training courses for counsellors in medical settings indicate the demand for specialist training. The part-time, one-year Diploma in Primary Health Care Counselling sponsored by the Counselling in Primary Care Trust, reflects its interest and involvement in promoting the development of training for counsellors in primary care. This course will cover models of brief therapy, teamworking in the NHS, models of health and illness, and personal and professional development. The British Association of Psychotherapists' one-year part time Counselling in General Practice course aims to provide a specialist training for counsellors in general practice but states that it will also be attractive to counsellors working in any multi-disciplinary health care setting. The objectives of this course are directed at some of the issues in general practice outlined in earlier chapters, in particular the interaction of psychosocial and physical factors in the aetiology and treatment of illness, group and organizational dynamics and working in a multi-disciplinary team. The infrastructure of training, qualifications and registration procedures required to underpin a cohesive, national system is growing organically in response to demand. This development needs to be coordinated and regulated if counselling in medical settings is to be recognized as a competent professional service.

SURFACE AND DEEP MESSAGES

Management of health care provision shows that it is possible, like some of the unfortunate victims of the Care in the Community Programme, to fall between the cracks of the said policies and the done policies. As in the linguistic structures that we use to describe policies, we attend to the deep structure, the meaning and implications, while we hear the surface structure of the words. The said message of a policy can stress collaboration and support. If this is merely political rhetoric which does not take account of practitioners' and users' views of their needs and priorities, it will be a hollow message, and bear little resemblance to what is actually done. The size of the gap between said and done policies can be used to give an indication of the measure of cynicism and despair felt by staff who have to implement new initiatives without adequate resources or support. The frustration caused by this tension is felt by Mariette, struggling to maintain her counselling role in a large hospital:

> statements of vision and mission are presented by management personnel, flushed with the excitement of re-entry after their latest course on Japanese style management, emphasising the

need to value and prize their staff and it's as if everything has been done, just in the saying of it.

Mariette's experiences illustrate the potential problem of introducing counselling into medical settings as a sop to public or popular demand when the reality is that it is an inadequately resourced provision, insufficient to meet actual need. *Health at Work in the NHS* might acknowledge the need for staff support and counselling while more traditional and entrenched habits, values and attitudes deny it, particularly if recognition of the need for support stigmatizes staff and affects their chances of promotion. Staff who cannot count themselves among those who need care because *they* are the carers express their needs in a language well understood and acceptable in medical settings. They get sick. Absences through staff sickness is estimated to cost the NHS as much as £200 million a year (HEA 1992).

The gap between said and done policy and practice is made most obvious when tragic stories about failures in community care hit the headlines. The same theme can be traced whenever mission statements promote intentions without adequate resources to follow them through. If the practice has to emphasize bottom-line results, the development of supportive relationships may be viewed as distractions which can be sacrificed to complete more quantitative targets. Much will ultimately depend on whether counselling and the training and support it requires is viewed as cost or investment in preventative care.

THE COSTS OF COUNSELLING

Recent advances in pharmacological treatments, especially when these are used in conjunction with other supportive measures, have enabled many people with severe depressive illnesses to function more effectively and get on with their lives. Counsellors need to be familiar with the arguments for and against the use of such treatments where there is a high risk of suicide and other violent and harmful behaviour linked to severe mental illnesses. Counselling or psychotherapy alone is unlikely to be an appropriate provision in such circumstances. However, the cost of prescribing enormous quantities of psychotropic drugs in the recent past, sometimes inappropriately, frequently for much longer than the precipitating need required, has been a major influence in the argument for counselling as a complementary provision.

The manufacture and distribution of drugs contributes towards the profits of the businesses that produce them and to their research, development and marketing. What profits are to be made from employing counsellors? We could count the savings to be made from the nation's drugs bill which could then be made more available to spend on a range of complementary treatments, including counselling. Another cost worth counting is human suffering. The consequences of causing mass addiction to benzodiazepines (minor tranquillizers), particularly in women, have been considerable (Walker 1990). The painful effects of withdrawal have raised awareness of over prescribing such drugs but the search for a panacea continues. This is not necessarily for alternative treatments and is more likely to be for improved drugs without unpleasant side-effects and addictive qualities. All of this happens alongside the work of substance misuse clinics, anti-drug campaigns for the young and horrific and frightening levels of inner-city drug problems.

Is the search for a designer drug that can be tailor-made to solve humanity's emotional problems the latest version of the search for the Holy Grail? There are enough actual historical antecedents, in addition to the religious, mythical and symbolic aspects, to demonstrate a drive towards finding single, unifying explanations that will enrich and transform our lives. The promise of counselling in medical settings with the offer of space and time to work through the feelings that underlie the symptoms, risks opening a Pandora's box of uncontainable feelings and demands that may contradict such an optimistic hope. Many people, women especially, visit their doctors for medical solutions to non-medical problems. They are not sick in their bodies but sick of their lives. Hence the need for counselling services as part of a supportive framework that includes appropriate medical treatment, health promotion clinics and self-help groups. The promotional appeal of counselling must be placed on the long-term benefits of enabling people to take care of themselves. This does not imply that counselling is the equivalent of drug treatments, with a compliance to a talking treatment instead of to a drug regime. All too easily this could become another way of masking pain to make the unbearable bearable. Counselling must be both a positive and a distinct alternative that mobilizes the 'healer in the patient' and is seen to do so. Counselling, as already stated, needs to take place within a context of appropriate choices.

Commercial interests and pressure groups concerned with profits are vastly more organized, purposeful and powerful than the pressure groups and individual voices demanding alternative treatments. Commercial groups have access to substantial resources to promote their products. It is also clear that powerful lobbies are at force in the allocations for funding to support major services such as the armed forces, health, education and social services. All these have well-established and integrated organizational structures and departments, ministries and secretaries of state. In the annual rounds of negotiations with the Treasury, each presents convincing arguments for plans to spend our money. Services which can present an impressive record in terms of action to make our lives safer and healthier are able to argue from a position of strength, especially when the general public has its expectations raised by the promise of new treatments and technology. The counselling services have less powerful lobbies. This is partly because their effectiveness is either long-term or largely unseen, except as complementary to other services. But it is also because the strength of the lobbying is diminished if the argument is not coherent, cohesive and linked to major political and political pressure groups. Decisions about what sort of society we live in are not determined by some abstract force for good – but by political will and strength. If counselling in medical settings has a future, as a healing process in its own right, its leaders will need to be able to take part in the political arenas where will is determined. In these circumstances being well-meaning is insufficient. Sophisticated political skills and strategies are needed in order to be heard and taken seriously.

EQUALITY

Access to counselling in medical settings is another example of the gap between the surface message and the deep structure of the provision, which is not available equally to everyone in the community. Daphne Wood's report for MIND (1993) states that there are about 100,000 people receiving psychotherapy in Britain, many of these in the NHS but others use a range of voluntary providers (Tyndall 1993), some of whom charge for their services, as well as independent practitioners (the latter restricting access to those who can pay). About one-third of general practices have counsellors or staff who take a counselling role. There are no current figures for the number of counsellors in hospitals, though the rising membership of the Counselling in Medical Settings Division of BAC gives some indication of an increase. People who are diagnosed as mentally ill or who present to their doctors with emotional and psychosocial problems are much more likely to be offered a physical rather than a talking treatment.

Although we can only roughly estimate the provision of counselling in medical settings we do know that, according to the BAC's
1993 membership survey, people have greater access to counsellors
if they live in the South-East of England. We have no clear picture of
who is getting what, nor is there at the time of writing any general
policy on the provision of counselling in medical settings. There is
evidence that 'certain groups of people . . . have less access to talking treatments than young, middle class, white heterosexuals' (Wood
1993:7). People with physical disabilities are frequently barred from
counselling provision because there are no counsellors in their area
in premises that are accessible. The same applies to non-English
speakers. Access is also limited if people do not have enough information about what is available. If there is confusion among the
providers, what hope for the clients? Greater availability of counselling and clear information about it could contribute towards people
having more choice and greater access to more appropriate provision at critical early stages, perhaps then avoiding eventual treatment with drugs and ECT. Users of services report their powerlessness
in choices about the availability and type of counselling and therapy
and therapists on offer (Wood 1993). The Marylebone Health Centre
(p. 65) is an example of a practice which has addressed many of
these issues. There are clear implications here for employers and
providers to confront these aspects. As training for counselling in
medical settings becomes more established, course providers will
need to address issues of access, equality and discrimination.

LOOKING TO THE FUTURE

Necessary questions about which therapies are most beneficial for
which people and how these should be made available are the
subject of ongoing research and evaluation. There has already been
a substantial amount of research into counselling in medical settings which has shown the benefits to be gained. It would be unfortunate if scarce resources were used to duplicate studies in the
name of reliability and at the expense of validity.

Medicine tends to attract people who need certainty and the 'right'
answers. A paradox is that they treat people but perhaps were
attracted to medicine via hard scientific subjects (physics/chemistry/
maths) which are still seen as entry qualifications to medical training. As a result the 'right' answers may be more attractive and
acceptable than exploration, and facts more appealing than ideas.
The ability to achieve grades in training which values memory and

getting answers right might predominate over the development of mature communication and interpersonal skills. This may intrinsically clash with a counselling ethos that embraces uncertainty and confusion, does not pretend to have answers for other people and sees few absolutes. Counselling tends to attract people who study arts and humanities and who are, on the whole, more centred on the whole person and more interested in the complexities of human relationships and needs.

The scientific method with its emphasis on objectivity, continues to dominate medical research including research into human relationships such as counselling. Yet modern physics has shown that the interaction of observer and observed is built into the nature of inquiry. Research methods that are rooted in the belief that subjective experience is an error to be eliminated are quite inappropriate for counselling. There has been some move away from hard-nosed objective research in recent years in areas such as education, but nevertheless the ethos of medicine is strongly scientific and consequently other methods of investigating subjective experience are still viewed with suspicion. Counselling is concerned precisely with the idea that the person is both subject and object and is able to reflect on experience. An important component of the relationship between counsellor and client is the counsellor's role as an observer of the client's intensely personal research that enables that person to find his or her own solutions. Counselling in medical settings is not something we give or do to our clients but is about offering opportunities for enabling relationships to develop which can help people to reach their own understanding and to find their own ways of coping with their experiences.

Although counselling in medical settings has many supporters among providers and clients it still has to justify its inclusion from within its context and respond to its detractors with proof of effectiveness. It is difficult to provide systematic, reliable and valid evidence of the effectiveness of a poorly resourced service that is still dependent on variously trained and qualified staff, many of whom work part-time. The findings of large-scale evaluative studies will provide valuable information in the future. In the meantime counsellors and employers need to work towards implementing guidelines such as those produced by BAC in order to establish counselling in medical settings as a professional service.

References

Abel-Smith, A., Irving, J. and Brown, P. (1989) Counselling in the medical context, in Dryden, W., Charles-Edwards, D. and Woolfe, R. *Handbook of Counselling in Great Britain*. London: Tavistock/Routledge.

Allen, L. (1989) A client's experience of failure, in Mearns, D. and Dryden, W. *Experiences of Counselling in Action*. London: Sage.

Anderson, S.A. and Hasler, J.C. (1979) Counselling in general practice. *Journal of the Royal College of Practitioners*, 29:352–6.

Ashurst, P.M. and Ward, D.F. (1983) *An Evaluation of Counselling in General Practice*. Final Report of the Leverhulme Counselling Project. London: Mental Health Foundation.

Argyle, M. (1972) *The Psychology of Interpersonal Behaviour*. Harmondsworth: Penguin Books.

Audit Commission (1986) *Making a Reality of Community Care*. London: HMSO.

Aveline, M. (1992) *From Medicine to Psychotherapy*. London: Whurr.

Balestrieri, M., Williams, P. and Wilkinson, G. (1988) Specialist mental health treatment in general practice: A meta-analysis. *Psychological Medicine*, 18:711–17.

Balint, E. and Norell, J.S. (1973) *Six Minutes for the Patient*. London: Tavistock.

Balint, E., Courtenay, M., Elder, A., Hull, S. and Julian, P. (1993) *The Doctor, The Patient and The Group: Balint Revisited*. London: Routledge.

Balint, M. (1957) *The Doctor, His Patient and the Illness*. London: Pitman.

Balint, M. (1989) *The Basic Fault: Therapeutic Aspects of Regression*. London: Tavistock/Routledge.

Blau, J.N. (1989) Time to let the patient speak. *British Medical Journal*, 298:39.

Bond, T. (1993) *Standards and Ethics for Counselling in Action*. London: Sage Publications.

Brandon, D. (1992) User power, in Barker, P. and Baldwin, S. (eds) *Ethical Issues in Mental Health*. London: Chapman Hall.

Breakwell, G.M. (1987) *Mapping Counselling in the Non-primary Sector of the NHS*, unpublished report for the British Association for Counselling.

Breggin, P.R. (1993) *Toxic Psychiatry: Drugs and Electroconvulsive Therapy – The Truth and the Better Alternatives.* London: Fontana.

Bridges, K. and Goldberg, D. (1985) Somatic presentation of DSM-III psychiatric disorders in primary care. *Journal of Psychosomatic Research*, 29, 563–9.

British Association for Counselling (1988) *Code of Ethics and Practice for the Supervision of Counsellors.* Rugby: BAC.

British Association for Counselling (1989) *Code of Ethics and Practice for Counselling Skills.* Rugby: BAC.

British Association for Counselling (1990) *Information Sheet 8 – Supervision.* Rugby: BAC.

British Association for Counselling National Register Working Party (UK) (1992) *Consultative Document: Proposal for a National Counselling Register.* Rugby: BAC.

British Association for Counselling (1993a) *Code of Ethics and Practice for Counsellors.* Rugby: BAC.

British Association for Counselling (1993b) *Guidelines for the Employment of Counsellors in General Practice.* Rugby: BAC.

Chambers, R. (1993) Avoiding burn-out in general practice. *British Journal of General Practice*, 43 (376):442.

Charlton, B. (1993) Holistic medicine or the humane doctor? *British Journal of General Practice*, 43 (376):475.

Cheshire, N., Knasel, E. and Davies, R. (1987) Self perception and individuation in children with psychosomatic pain, in Cheshire, N. and Thomae, H. (eds) *Self, Symptoms and Psychotherapy.* Chichester: John Wiley and Sons Ltd.

Clothier, Sir C. (1994) *The Allitt Inquiry.* London: HMSO.

Corney, R.H. (1990) Counselling in general practice – does it work? Discussion paper, *Journal of Social Medicine*, 83:253–7.

Corney, R. (1993) Studies of the effectiveness of counselling in general practice, in Corney, R.H. and Jenkins, R. (eds) *Counselling in General Practice.* London: Tavistock/Routledge.

Corney, R.H. and Jenkins, R. (eds) (1993) *Counselling in General Practice.* London: Tavistock/Routledge.

Curran, A. and Higgs, R. (1993) Setting up a counsellor in primary care: The evolution and experience in one general practice, in Corney, R.H. and Jenkins, R. (eds) *Counselling in General Practice.* London: Tavistock/Routledge.

Department of Health (1989) *Caring For People: Community Care into the Next Decade and Beyond.* Cmnd. 849. London: HMSO.

Department of Health (1990) *Caring For People: Policy Guidelines.* London: HMSO.

Department of Health (1991) *The Patient's Charter.* London: HMSO.

Department of Health (1992) *The Health of the Nation.* Cmnd. 1523. London: HMSO.

Department of Health (1993) *The Health of the Nation: Key Area Handbook on Mental Illness.* London: HMSO.

Department of Health (in press) *Defeat Depression: Management Guidelines,* London: HMSO. (For further information please contact the Administrator of the Defeat Depression Campaign c/o Royal College of Psychiatrists, 17 Belgrave Square, London SW1X 8PG.)

DHSS (1986) *Neighbourhood Nursing: A Focus for Care.* Report of the Community Nursing Review (Chair Julia Cumberlege), London: HMSO.

DHSS (1986) *Primary Health Care: An Agenda for Discussion.* Cmnd. 9771. London: HMSO.

Derbyshire FHSA (1994) *Guidelines for the Employment of Counsellors in Primary Care.* Derwent Court, Stuart Street, Derby. DE1 2FZ.

Ditchfield, H. (1992) 'The birth of a child with mental handicap:' Coping with loss, in Waitman, A. and Conboy Hill, S. (eds) *Psychotherapy and Mental Handicap.* London: Sage Publications.

Dryden, W. (ed.) (1984) *Individual Therapies in Britain.* London: Harper and Row.

Dryden, W., Charles-Edwards, D. and Woolfe, R. (eds) (1989) *Handbook of Counselling in Great Britain.* London: Tavistock/Routledge in association with BAC.

East, P.I. (1995) The mentoring relationship, in Ellis, R.B., Gates, R. and Kenworthy, N. *Interpersonal Communication in Nursing.* Edinburgh: Churchill Livingstone.

Fitzgerald, P. (1994) Counselling in practice. *Health Director:* June: 13

Freeling, P., Rao, B.M., Paykel, E.S. (1985) Unrecognised depression in general practice. *British Medical Journal,* 290:1880–3.

Gask, L., McGrath, G., Goldberg, D. and Millar, T. (1987) Improving the psychiatric skills of established general practitioners: Evaluation of group teaching. *Medical Education,* 21:362–8.

Gask, L., Brandman, J. and Standart, S. (1991) Teaching communication skills: A problem based approach. *Postgraduate Education for General Practice,* 2:7–15.

Goffman, E. (1961) *Asylums: Essays on the Social Situation of Mental Patients and Other Inmates.* Harmondsworth: Penguin.

Goldberg, D. and Huxley, P. (1992) *Common mental disorders: A biosocial model.* London: Tavistock/Routledge.

Goldie, L. (1986) Psychoanalysis in the National Health Service General Hospital, *Psychoanalytical Psychology,* 1 (2):23–34.

Göpfert, M. and Barnes, B. (1994) *Counsellors and Secondary Mental Health Care* (Unpublished presentation) Liverpool Psychotherapy and Consultation Service.

Griffiths, R. (1988) *Community Care: Agenda for Action.* London: HMSO.

Groddeck, G. (1977) *The Meaning of Illness.* London: The Hogarth Press and The Institute of Psychoanalysis.

Groves, T. (ed.) (1993) *Countdown to Community Care.* London: BMJ Publications.

Guggenbuhl-Craig, A. (1979) *Power in the Helping Professions.* Irving, TX: Spring Publications.

Hasler, J. (1993) The primary health care teams: History and contractual farces, in Pringle, M. (ed.) *Change and Teamwork in Primary Care*. London: BMJ Publishing Group.

Health Education Authority (1992) *Health at Work in the NHS Action Pack*. London: Health Education Authority.

Healy, D. (1990) *The Suspended Revolution: Psychiatry and Psychotherapy Re-examined*. London: Faber and Faber.

Hobson, R.E. (1985) *Forms of Feeling: The Heart of Psychotherapy*. London: Tavistock/Routledge.

Holdsworth, A. (1988) *Out of the Dolls House. The Story of Women in the Twentieth Century*. London: BBC Books.

Howard, L.M. and Wessely, S. (1993) The psychology of multiple allergy. *British Medical Journal*, 307:747–8.

Hurd, J. and Rowland, N. (1991) *Counselling in General Practice, A Guide for Counsellors*, revised edn. Rugby: British Association for Counselling.

Ignatieff, M. (1994) *Scar Tissue*. London: Vintage.

Irving, J. and Heath, V. (1989) *Counselling in General Practice: A Guide for General Practitioners*, revised edn. Rugby: British Association for Counselling.

Ives, G. (1979) Psychological treatment in general practice. *Journal of the Royal College of Practitioners*, 29:343–51.

Jacobs, M. (1984) Psychodynamic therapy: The Freudian approach, in Dryden, W. (ed.) *Individual Therapy in Britain*. London: Harper and Row.

Jenkins, R. and Gillon, R. (1993) The ethics of counselling, in Corney, R. and Jenkins, R. (eds) *Counselling in General Practice*. London: Routledge.

Kahtan, S. and Fitton, P. (1993) Listen to me. *British Medical Journal*, 307:571.

King, M. (1994) Counselling services in general practice: The need for evaluation. *Psychiatric Bulletin*, 18:65–7.

King, M., Broster, G., and Horder, J. (1994) Controlled trials in the evaluation of counselling in general practice. *British Journal of General Practice*, 44:229–32.

King's Fund Commission (1992) *Londoners' Views on the Future of Health Care – An Interim Report for the King's Fund Commission on the Future of Acute Health Services*. London Research Centre.

Klein, R. (1993) Dimensions of rationing: Who should do what?. *British Medical Journal*, 307:309–11.

Kübler-Ross, E. (1989) *On Death and Dying*. London: Routledge.

Kuhn, T.S. (1962) *The Structure of Scientific Revolutions*. Chicago, IL: University of Chicago Press.

Laing, R.D. (1967) *The Politics of Experience*. Harmondsworth: Penguin Books.

Lawrence, M. (1993) Caring for the future, in Pringle, M. (ed.) *Change and Teamwork in Primary Care*. London: BMJ Publishing Group.

McDougal, J. (1986) *Theatres of the Mind: Illusion and Truth on the Psychoanalytic Stage*. London: Free Association Books.

McDougal, J. (1989) *Theatres of the Body: A Psychoanalytic Approach to Psychosomatic Illness*. London: Free Association Books.

Main, T. (1957) The ailment. *British Journal of Medical Psychology*, 30:129–45.

Mann, A. (1993) The need for counselling, in Corney, R. and Jenkins, R. (eds) *Counselling in General Practice*. London: Tavistock/Routledge.

Marks, J.N., Goldberg, D.P. and Hillier, V.F. (1979) Determinants of the ability of general practitioners to detect psychiatric illness. *Psychological Medicine*, 9:337–53.

Markus, A.C., Murray Parkes, C., Tomson, P. and Johnston, M. (1989) *Psychological Problems in General Practice*. Oxford: Oxford University Press.

Marsh, G.N. and Barr, J. (1975) Marriage guidance counselling in a group practice. *Journal of the Royal College of Practitioners*, 25:73–5.

Martin, C. (1993) Attached, detached or new recruits? in Pringle, M. (ed.) *Change and Teamwork in Primary Care*. London: BMJ Publishing Group.

Martin, E. (1988) Counselling in General Practice. *British Medical Journal*, 297:637–8.

Martin, E. and Martin, P.M.L. (1985) Changes in psychological diagnosis and prescription in a practice employing a counsellor. *Family Practice*, (2) 4:241–3.

Martin, E. and Mitchell, H. (1983) A counsellor in general practice: a one-year survey. *Journal of the Royal College of General Practitioners*, 33:366–7.

Masson, J.M. (1989) *Against Therapy*. London: Harper Collins.

Menzies, I. (1961) *The Functioning of Social Systems as a Defence Against Anxiety*. London: Tavistock.

Menzies-Lyth, I. (1988) *Containing Anxiety in Institutions*. London: Free Association Books.

MIND (1993) *Policy Pack*. London: MIND Publications.

NHS Management Executive (1990) *Nursing in the Community*. London: North West Thames Regional Health Authority.

Noon, J.M. (1992) Counselling general practitioners: The scope and limitation of the medical role in counselling. *Journal of the Royal Society of Medicine*, 85:126–8.

Norton, M. (1958) *The Borrowers*. Harmondsworth: Penguin Books.

Parry, G. (1994) From research to care: Modifying treatment in the light of research, *Collaboration in Care*, *Proceedings of the 3rd St. George's Counselling in Primary Care Conference*, London: St. George's Mental Health Library Conference Series.

Petterson, G. (1992) User views on counselling services provided at the Forest Hill Road Group Practice. *CMS News*, 32:1–4.

Pietroni, P.C. (1993) Beyond the boundaries: Relationship between general practice and complementary medicine, in Pringle, M. (ed.) *Change and Teamwork in Primary Care*. London: BMJ Publishing Group.

Pringle, M. (ed.) (1993) *Change and Teamwork in Primary Care*. London: BMJ Publishing Group.

Rawnsley, K. (1991) The national counselling service for sick doctors. *Proceedings of the Royal College of Physicians of Edinburgh*, (21):1.

Rippere, V. (1987) Environmental factors in anxiety states. *CMS News*, 13:12–17.

Rogers, A. and Pilgrim, D. (1993) Mental Health Service users' views of medical practitioners. *Journal of Interprofessional Care*, June.

Rowland, N., Irving, J. and Maynard, A. (1989) Can general practitioners counsel? *Journal of the Royal College of Practitioners*, 39:118–20.

Scott, M.G.B. and Marinker, M. (1993) Imposed change in general practice, in Pringle, M. (ed.) *Change and Teamwork in Primary Care*. London: BMJ Publishing Group.

Seale, C. and Pattison, S. (eds) (1994) *Medical Knowledge: Doubt and Certainty*. Buckingham: Open University Press.

Secretaries of State for Social Services, Wales, Northern Ireland and Scotland (1987) *Promoting Better Health*. Cmnd. 249. London: HMSO.

Secretaries of State for Social Services, Wales, Northern Ireland and Scotland (1989) *Working for Patients*, London: HMSO.

Sharpe, E.F. (1940) An examination of metaphors, in Sharpe, E.F. (1950) *Collected Papers*. London: Hogarth Press.

Sheldon, M. (1992) *Counselling in General Practice*. Exeter: Royal College of General Practitioners.

Sheppard, J. (1993) The clinical task, in Pringle, M. (ed.) *Change and Teamwork in Primary Care*. London: BMJ Publishing Group.

Sibbald, B., Addington-Hall, J., Brenneman, D. and Freeling, P. (1993) Counsellors in English and Welsh general practices: Their nature and distribution. *British Medical Journal*, 306:29–33.

Skynner, R. and Cleese, J. (1983) *Families and How to Survive Them*. London: Methuen.

Sontag, S. (1978) *Illness as Metaphor*. Harmondsworth: Penguin Books.

Sontag, S. (1991) *Illness as Metaphor: Aids and its Metaphors*. Harmondsworth: Penguin Books

Strathdee, G. and Sutherby, D. (1993) *Literature Review for the Development of a Primary Care Strategy for Mental Health*, Prism (Psychiatric Research in Service Measurement), London: Institute of Psychiatry.

Sturgeon, D. (1985) Medical student training: The situation in Great Britain, in Wolff, H.H., Knaus, W. and Brautigam, W. (eds) *First Steps in Psychotherapy: Teaching Psychotherapy to Medical Students and General Practitioners*. Berlin: Springer-Verlag.

Syme, G. (1993) *Counselling in Independent Practice*. Buckingham: Open University Press.

Symington, N. (1992) Counter-transference with mentally handicapped clients, in Waitman, A. and Conboy Hill, S. (eds) *Psychotherapy and Mental Handicap*. London: Sage.

Szaz, T. (1974) *The Myth of Mental Illness: Foundations of a Theory of Personal Conduct*. New York: Harper Row.

Thomas, R.V.R. and Corney, R.H. (1993) Working with community health professionals: A survey among general practitioners. *British Journal of General Practice*, 43 (375):417–21.

Tylee, A.T., Freeling, P. and Kerry, S. (1993) Why do general practitioners recognize major depression in one woman patient yet miss it in another? *The British Journal of General Practice*, 43 (373):327–30.

Tyndall, N. (1993) *Counselling in the Voluntary Sector*. Buckingham: Open University Press.

Tyrer, P., Higgs, R. and Strathdee, G. (1993) *Mental Health and Primary Care: A Changing Agenda*. London: Gaskell and the Mental Health Foundation.

UKCC (1986) *Project 2000: A New Preparation for Practice*. London: UKCC.

Waitman, A. and Conboy Hill, S. (1992) *Psychotherapy and Mental Handicap*. London: Sage.

Walker, M. (1990) *Women in Therapy and Counselling*. Buckingham: Open University Press.

Warner, R.W., Gater, R., Jackson, M.G. and Goldberg, D.P. (1993) Effects of a community mental health service on the practice and attitudes of general practitioners. *British Journal of General Practice*, 34 (377):507–11.

Waydenfeld, D. and Waydenfeld, S.W. (1980) Counselling in general practice. *Journal of the Royal College of General Practitioners*, 30:671–7.

Williams, J., Watson, G., Smith, H., Copperman, J. and Wood, D. (1993) *Purchasing Effective Mental Health Services for Women: A Framework For Action*. London: MIND Publications.

Winnicott, D.W. (1971) *Playing and Reality*. New York: Basic Books.

Winnicott, D.W. (1990) *Maturational Processes and the Facilitating Environment*. London: Karnac Books and the Institute of Psychoanalysis.

Wolff, H.H., Knaus, W. and Brautigam, W. (eds) (1985) *First Steps in Psychotherapy. Teaching Psychotherapy to Medical Students and General Practitioners*. Berlin: Springer-Verlag.

Wood, D. (1993) *Wordswordswordswords, the Power of Words: Uses and Abuses of Talking Treatments*. London: MIND Publications.

Index

References in italic indicate figures or tables.

COUNSELLING FOR WOMEN

Janet Perry

Although few in number, organizations which provide counselling services for women have had a tremendous impact on our current understanding of women's psychology and the issues women explore in counselling. Through her examination of these organizations, Janet Perry highlights the unique emphasis they place on the importance of how services are provided and their exploration of the dynamics of the working relationships of women counsellors. The organizations included in the book range from Women's Aid to Women's Therapy Centres and their services are considered in the context of counselling women. The study shows that through a self-reflexive examination of their organizational processes, these agencies have come to a greater understanding of the ways in which women working with women create non-hierarchical and cooperative endeavours, much needed in our individualistic and competitive society. The book illustrates the conflicts that arise when both modes seek to exist within one organization – Family Service Units – and the struggle all the agencies have to legitimize these ways of working to a male dominated system from which funding is often sought. Recommended reading for all those involved in counselling and psychotherapy, this book illustrates some of the practical outcomes of these alternative working models.

Contents
The development of counselling in women's organizations – Counselling in women's organizations – The practice of counselling women – Specific issues in counselling women – Professional relationships in counselling for women – Critique of counselling for women – References – Index.

128pp   0 335 19034 0 (Paperback)

COUNSELLING IN THE VOLUNTARY SECTOR
Nicholas Tyndall

Nicholas Tyndall has drawn upon his extensive experience of counselling and training in personal and family organizations to provide a comprehensive picture of the voluntary sector. In his clear, accessible style, he outlines the beginnings of counselling in Britain and charts the development of the growing number of specialist and generic agencies.

The book is written in the firm belief that the voluntary sector can combine what is best in the amateur and the professional. Its scope and practices are explored. Methods of selection, training and supervision of counsellors are compared, and the challenges facing staff and management committees are examined. The book highlights the strengths and weaknesses of voluntary counselling, and identifies the need to improve equal opportunities, fill new gaps and develop inter-agency collaboration. The author has harsh words for public bodies which have high expectations of volunteers but are not prepared to meet the cost. He offers helpful advice for existing agencies and those wanting to improve their personal services; and guidance to individuals who are interested in becoming counsellors.

Contents
The development of counselling in the voluntary sector – Voluntary agencies – The practice of counselling in the voluntary sector – Specific issues in counselling in the voluntary sector – Professional relationships in counselling in the voluntary sector – A critique of counselling in the voluntary sector – References – Index.

160pp   0 335 19027 8 (Paperback)